WHAT TO EXPECT WHEN EXPECTING A BABY

PREGNANCY GUIDE

AMANDA WILLIAMS

TABLE OF CONTENTS

POSTPARTUM RECOVERY
- Physical recovery for moms
- Emotional adjustments
- Support networks and postpartum care

PARENTING TIPS
- Bonding with your baby
- Balancing work and family
- Childproofing and safety measures

FINANCIAL PLANNING
- Budgeting for a new arrival
- Planning for parental leave

INTRODUCTION TO PREGNANCY

THE JOURNEY

Pregnancy is a transformative and multifaceted journey that encompasses physical, emotional, and psychological changes for both the expecting mother and her partner. This remarkable process typically spans around 40 weeks, divided into three trimesters. Each trimester unfolds with its own set of developments and challenges, contributing to the overall growth and preparation for the arrival of a new life.

In the first trimester, the initial sense of elation and anticipation is often accompanied by physical manifestations such as morning sickness, heightened sensitivity to certain smells, and fatigue. The body undergoes crucial developments during this period, with the formation of vital organs and the initial stages of fetal growth. Emotionally, expectant parents may experience a mix of excitement and anxiety as they come to terms with the impending changes in their lives.

As the journey progresses into the second trimester, many women find relief from early pregnancy symptoms. This period is often referred to as the "honeymoon phase" of pregnancy, characterized by increased energy levels and a visible baby bump. During this time, prenatal care becomes even more critical, with regular check-ups, ultrasounds, and screenings to monitor both maternal and fetal well-being. Expectant parents may start feeling the baby's movements, fostering a deeper connection with the growing life within.

The third trimester, marked by the final stretch of pregnancy, brings its own set of challenges. The physical demands on the mother intensify as the baby continues to grow, leading to increased discomfort, difficulty sleeping, and heightened emotions. Preparations for labor and delivery become more tangible, with childbirth education classes, creating birth plans, and packing hospital bags. This period is also characterized by the baby settling into a head-down position, getting ready for the journey into the world.

Throughout the entire journey, open communication between partners is essential. As the body undergoes significant changes, emotional support becomes paramount. Expecting parents may share in the joy of hearing the baby's heartbeat during ultrasound appointments and may also encounter the need for flexibility and adaptability as unexpected challenges arise.

Ultimately, the journey of pregnancy is a unique and awe-inspiring experience that brings with it a mix of emotions, physical transformations, and the promise of new beginnings. It is a time of anticipation, preparation, and profound connection, laying the foundation for the incredible adventure that awaits with the birth of a child.

UNDERSTANDING THE TRIMESTERS

Pregnancy is a complex and dynamic process that unfolds over approximately 40 weeks, commonly divided into three trimesters. Each trimester is characterized by distinct developmental milestones for both the mother and the growing fetus. This extended period allows for a comprehensive journey of gestation, enabling the gradual formation and maturation of essential structures that pave the way for a healthy newborn.

First Trimester: Weeks 1-12

The first trimester is a critical phase marked by the initial stages of conception and the formation of the early embryo. In the first few weeks, fertilization of the egg by sperm leads to the creation of a single-cell zygote. This zygote undergoes rapid cell division, forming a blastocyst that implants itself into the uterine lining. As the weeks progress, the blastocyst transforms into an embryo, and the basic structures of the body begin to take shape.

One of the hallmark events of the first trimester is the development of the neural tube, which eventually becomes the brain and spinal cord. Simultaneously, the heart starts to beat, and the circulatory system takes form. Basic facial features, limbs, and major internal organs begin to develop, laying the foundation for the intricate network of systems that will sustain life outside the womb.

For the expectant mother, the first trimester often brings a mix of emotions and physical changes. Hormonal fluctuations can contribute to symptoms such as morning sickness, heightened sense of smell, and fatigue. The body undergoes adaptations to support the growing fetus, with increased blood volume and changes in the uterus and placenta.

Despite the challenges, the first trimester is a period of anticipation and discovery. The confirmation of pregnancy through home pregnancy tests or medical examinations often marks the beginning of a new chapter for expectant parents. Prenatal care becomes a focal point during this trimester, with initial check-ups, screenings, and discussions about nutrition and lifestyle choices.

Second Trimester: Weeks 13-26

The second trimester is commonly considered the "honeymoon phase" of pregnancy. Many women experience a relief from the early symptoms of morning sickness, and energy levels often rise. This trimester is characterized by visible changes in the mother's body, as the baby bump becomes more pronounced.

By the beginning of the second trimester, most of the critical fetal structures are in place, and the focus shifts to growth and refinement. The fetus goes through a period of rapid development, with the bones ossifying, muscles strengthening, and the reproductive organs becoming distinguishable. The skin develops a protective layer called vernix, and fine hair known as lanugo covers the body.

Around the midpoint of pregnancy, typically during week 20, many expectant parents undergo an ultrasound that allows them to see their baby's anatomy and possibly determine the gender. Feeling the baby's movements, known as "quickening," becomes a significant milestone, fostering a tangible connection between parents and their unborn child.

Prenatal care remains crucial during the second trimester, with regular check-ups to monitor the health of both the mother and the developing fetus. Various screenings, such as the anatomy scan and glucose tolerance test, are commonly performed during this period to identify any potential issues.

Emotionally, the second trimester often brings a sense of joy and anticipation. With the physical discomforts of the first trimester alleviated, many women find this time to be particularly enjoyable. Partners may become more actively involved in the pregnancy, attending appointments and feeling the baby's movements. It is also a period for expectant parents to start preparing for the impending arrival, considering baby names, creating a nursery, and attending childbirth education classes.

Third Trimester: Weeks 27-40

The third trimester encompasses the final stretch of pregnancy, characterized by the continuing growth and maturation of the fetus. This phase presents unique challenges for both the mother and the baby, as the body undergoes significant changes in preparation for labor and delivery.

As the baby gains weight and accumulates more body fat, the mother may experience increased physical discomfort. Common symptoms include backache, swollen ankles, and difficulty sleeping. The baby's movements, which were initially subtle, become more pronounced and may even cause discomfort. The third trimester is also marked by the descent of the baby into the pelvis, preparing for the birthing process.

Prenatal care remains a priority, with more frequent check-ups to monitor the baby's position, growth, and the overall health of the mother. Some expectant parents opt for additional prenatal classes focused on labor and delivery, providing valuable information and support as the due date approaches.

Emotionally, the third trimester can be a mix of excitement and apprehension. As the baby's arrival becomes imminent, parents may experience a range of emotions, from joy and anticipation to anxiety about labor and the challenges of parenthood. It is a time for finalizing birth plans, packing the hospital bag, and ensuring that all preparations are in place for the homecoming of the newborn.

The culmination of the third trimester is the onset of labor, leading to the miraculous moment of childbirth. The birthing process involves a series of contractions, cervical dilation, and ultimately, the delivery of the baby. The support of healthcare professionals, birthing partners, and a well-prepared birth plan can contribute to a positive birthing experience.

Understanding the trimesters of pregnancy provides a comprehensive insight into the intricate journey of gestation. From the initial moments of conception to the final stages of preparation for labor, each trimester brings its own set of challenges and milestones. This gradual progression allows for the optimal development of the fetus and the physical and emotional readiness of expectant parents for the transformative experience of bringing a new life into the world.

NUTRITION AND PRENATAL CARE

HEALTHY EATING DURING PREGNANCY

Pregnancy is a time of significant physiological changes, and proper nutrition is crucial to support the health and development of both the expectant mother and the growing fetus. A well-balanced and nutrient-rich diet during pregnancy provides essential vitamins, minerals, and energy, contributing to optimal fetal growth, maternal well-being, and the prevention of potential complications.

Nutritional Requirements During Pregnancy:

The nutritional needs during pregnancy are unique, requiring careful attention to ensure the adequate intake of key nutrients. While the precise requirements may vary for each individual, there are general guidelines that can serve as a foundation for a healthy pregnancy diet.

Folic Acid:
Folic acid is crucial in the early stages of pregnancy for preventing neural tube defects in the developing fetus. Sources include leafy green vegetables, fortified cereals, beans, and citrus fruits.

Iron:
Iron is essential for the production of hemoglobin and
the prevention of anemia in both the mother and the
baby.
Good sources of iron include lean meats, poultry, fish,
beans, and fortified cereals.

Calcium:
Calcium is vital for the development of the baby's bones
and teeth and is also important for the mother's bone
health.
Dairy products, leafy green vegetables, and fortified
plant-based milk are excellent sources.

Protein:
Protein is crucial for the development of the baby's
organs, muscles, and tissues.
Good sources include lean meats, poultry, fish, eggs,
dairy products, legumes, and nuts.

Omega-3 Fatty Acids:
Omega-3 fatty acids, particularly DHA, play a role in the
development of the baby's brain and eyes.
Fatty fish, chia seeds, flaxseeds, and walnuts are rich
sources.

Vitamin D:
Vitamin D is essential for the absorption of calcium and
the development of the baby's bones.
Sun exposure, fortified foods, and supplements are
common sources.

Iodine:
Iodine is crucial for the development of the baby's brain and nervous system.
Seafood, dairy products, and iodized salt are good sources.

Vitamin C:
Vitamin C enhances iron absorption and supports the immune system.
Citrus fruits, strawberries, bell peppers, and broccoli are rich in vitamin C.

Balanced Diet and Meal Planning:

Achieving a well-balanced diet during pregnancy involves incorporating a variety of nutrient-dense foods into daily meals. A diverse and colorful plate ensures the intake of a broad spectrum of vitamins and minerals. Here are some guidelines for creating a balanced diet during pregnancy:

Fruits and Vegetables:
Aim for a variety of colorful fruits and vegetables to obtain a range of vitamins, minerals, and antioxidants.
Include leafy greens, berries, citrus fruits, carrots, and cruciferous vegetables in your diet.

Whole Grains:
Choose whole grains such as brown rice, quinoa, oats, and whole wheat bread for fiber, B vitamins, and sustained energy.

Protein Sources:
Include a mix of lean meats, poultry, fish, eggs, dairy products, legumes, and plant-based protein sources like tofu and tempeh.

Dairy or Alternatives:
Ensure an adequate intake of calcium through dairy products or fortified plant-based alternatives like almond milk or soy milk.

Healthy Fats:
Incorporate sources of healthy fats such as avocados, nuts, seeds, and olive oil for essential fatty acids and overall well-being.

Hydration:
Drink plenty of water to stay hydrated, support digestion, and help prevent constipation.

Foods to Limit or Avoid:

While focusing on nutrient-dense foods, it's also important to be mindful of foods that may pose risks during pregnancy. Certain foods should be limited or avoided to minimize potential harm to the developing fetus:

Raw or Undercooked Seafood and Meat:
To prevent foodborne illnesses, avoid raw or undercooked seafood and meats.

High-Mercury Fish:
Limit the consumption of high-mercury fish like shark, swordfish, king mackerel, and tilefish.

Unpasteurized Dairy and Soft Cheeses:
Avoid unpasteurized dairy products and soft cheeses like feta, Brie, and blue cheese, as they may carry the risk of bacterial contamination.

Caffeine:
Limit caffeine intake to moderate levels (usually 200-300 mg per day) to reduce the risk of preterm birth and low birth weight.

Alcohol:
Abstain from alcohol, as it can have detrimental effects on fetal development.

Processed and High-Sugar Foods:
Minimize the consumption of processed foods and foods high in added sugars, as they offer little nutritional value.

Nutritional Supplements:

In addition to obtaining nutrients from food, prenatal supplements may be recommended to ensure adequate intake, especially for certain vitamins and minerals. Common prenatal supplements include:

Folic Acid or Folate:
Often prescribed before conception and during the first trimester to prevent neural tube defects.

Iron:
Recommended to prevent iron-deficiency anemia.

Calcium:
If dietary intake is insufficient, calcium supplements may be recommended.

Vitamin D:
Especially important for individuals with limited sun exposure.

Omega-3 Fatty Acids:
For those who don't consume sufficient fatty fish, supplements can provide essential omega-3s.
It's crucial to consult with healthcare professionals before starting any supplement regimen to ensure individualized and appropriate recommendations.

Lifestyle Considerations:

Apart from dietary choices, certain lifestyle considerations can contribute to a healthy and fulfilling pregnancy:

Regular Exercise:

Engage in moderate exercise, such as walking, swimming, or prenatal yoga, to support overall health and well-being.

Adequate Rest:
Ensure sufficient rest and quality sleep to promote physical and emotional well-being.

Stress Management:
Practice stress-reducing techniques, such as meditation or deep breathing exercises, to promote a calm and positive mindset.

Regular Prenatal Check-ups:
Attend regular prenatal check-ups to monitor both maternal and fetal health.

Avoiding Harmful Substances:
Steer clear of smoking, recreational drugs, and exposure to harmful chemicals to protect the developing fetus.

Healthy eating during pregnancy is a cornerstone of maternal and fetal well-being, providing the essential nutrients necessary for optimal growth and development. A well-balanced diet, rich in a variety of nutrient-dense foods, along with appropriate supplements.

PRENATAL VITAMIN AND SUPPLEMENTS

Pregnancy is a transformative journey that places unique demands on a woman's body. To support the health and development of both the expectant mother and the growing fetus, prenatal vitamins and supplements play a crucial role.

Why Prenatal Vitamins?

Prenatal vitamins are specially formulated supplements designed to meet the increased nutritional needs of pregnant women. While a well-balanced diet is the foundation of a healthy pregnancy, prenatal vitamins act as a nutritional safety net, ensuring that both the mother and the developing baby receive essential nutrients in adequate amounts. The decision to take prenatal vitamins is often recommended by healthcare professionals and is based on factors such as dietary habits, individual nutritional requirements, and potential risk factors.

Key Nutrients in Prenatal Vitamins:

Folic Acid (Folate):
Folic acid is a critical nutrient, especially in the early stages of pregnancy, as it helps prevent neural tube defects in the developing fetus.
Adequate folate intake is crucial before conception and during the first trimester when the neural tube is forming.

Iron:

Iron is essential for preventing iron-deficiency anemia in both the mother and the baby.
During pregnancy, the body's demand for iron increases significantly to support the expansion of blood volume and the growing fetus.

Calcium:
Calcium is vital for the development of the baby's bones and teeth and is also important for the mother's bone health.
Insufficient calcium intake may lead to the body extracting calcium from the mother's bones, potentially resulting in bone density issues.

Vitamin D:
Vitamin D is crucial for the absorption of calcium and plays a role in the development of the baby's bones.
Adequate vitamin D is necessary to ensure the proper utilization of calcium for both the mother and the baby.

Omega-3 Fatty Acids (DHA):
Omega-3 fatty acids, particularly DHA (docosahexaenoic acid), are essential for the development of the baby's brain and eyes.
Adequate DHA intake during pregnancy is associated with improved cognitive development in the offspring.

Iodine:
Iodine is crucial for the development of the baby's brain and nervous system.

Insufficient iodine intake during pregnancy can lead to cognitive impairments in the baby.

Vitamin C:
Vitamin C enhances iron absorption and supports the immune system.
Adequate vitamin C intake helps address iron-deficiency anemia, a common concern during pregnancy.

Zinc:
Zinc is important for fetal growth and development and is essential for various cellular processes.
Inadequate zinc levels during pregnancy may contribute to complications such as low birth weight.

Vitamin B12:
Vitamin B12 is essential for the formation of red blood cells and the development of the nervous system.
Adequate B12 intake is particularly important for mothers following vegetarian or vegan diets, as this vitamin is primarily found in animal products.

Choosing the Right Prenatal Vitamin:

Selecting an appropriate prenatal vitamin involves considering individual nutritional needs, dietary restrictions, and potential risk factors. Here are some factors to consider when choosing a prenatal vitamin:

Folic Acid Content:

Ensure that the prenatal vitamin contains the recommended amount of folic acid (usually around 400-800 micrograms).
Some women may require higher doses, so individualized recommendations from healthcare professionals are valuable.

Iron Formulation:
Choose a prenatal vitamin with a form of iron that is easily absorbed, such as ferrous bisglycinate or iron citrate.
Iron supplements are often needed, especially in the later stages of pregnancy, to prevent iron-deficiency anemia.

Calcium and Vitamin D Levels:
Check the levels of calcium and vitamin D in the prenatal vitamin, but be aware that additional supplementation may be necessary, depending on dietary intake and sun exposure.

Omega-3 Fatty Acids:
Consider prenatal vitamins that include DHA, or opt for a separate omega-3 supplement to ensure adequate intake.

Iodine Inclusion:
Ensure that the prenatal vitamin contains iodine, as this is crucial for the development of the baby's brain and nervous system.

Compatibility with Dietary Restrictions:
If following a vegetarian or vegan diet, verify that the prenatal vitamin is free from animal-derived ingredients.
Individuals with specific allergies or sensitivities should carefully review the ingredients of prenatal vitamins.

Doctor's Recommendations:
Always consult with healthcare professionals, such as obstetricians or midwives, for personalized advice on prenatal vitamin selection.

Supplementing Safely:

While prenatal vitamins are generally considered safe, it's important to use them as directed and not exceed recommended dosages. Excessive intake of certain vitamins and minerals can have adverse effects. Here are some additional considerations for safe supplementation:

Avoiding Overdosing:
Excessive vitamin A intake, particularly in the form of retinol, can lead to birth defects.
Choose prenatal vitamins with a safe level of vitamin A and avoid additional high-dose vitamin A supplements.

Iron Supplementation:
Iron supplements may cause constipation, nausea, or stomach upset. Taking them with food or choosing a

slow-release formulation can help minimize these side effects.

Nausea and Timing:
If prenatal vitamins contribute to nausea, try taking them with a meal or at bedtime.
Splitting the dose throughout the day can also help enhance absorption and reduce stomach discomfort.

Interaction with Other Medications:
Inform healthcare professionals about any other supplements or medications being taken, as certain combinations may lead to interactions.

Monitoring Vitamin D Levels:
Regularly check vitamin D levels, especially for individuals with limited sun exposure, to determine if additional supplementation is necessary.

Addressing Dietary Gaps:

While prenatal vitamins are valuable, they should complement, not substitute, a healthy and balanced diet. Whole foods offer a wide array of nutrients and bioactive compounds that supplements cannot fully replicate. Here are some tips for addressing dietary gaps during pregnancy:

Emphasize Nutrient-Dense Foods:
Focus on whole, nutrient-dense foods such as fruits, vegetables, whole grains, lean proteins, and healthy fats.

Diversify Protein Sources:
Incorporate a variety of protein sources, including lean meats, poultry, fish, eggs, dairy products, legumes, and plant-based options.

Include Omega-3-Rich Foods:
Consume fatty fish, chia seeds, flaxseeds, and walnuts to enhance omega-3 fatty acid intake.

Calcium-Rich Choices:
Include dairy products, fortified plant-based milks, leafy greens, and almonds to support calcium needs.

REGULAR CHECK-UPS AND SCREENINGS

Pregnancy is a transformative journey marked by numerous milestones, and regular check-ups and screenings play a pivotal role in ensuring the well-being of both the expectant mother and the developing fetus. These medical evaluations, conducted by healthcare professionals, monitor the progress of pregnancy, identify potential complications, and provide essential information for informed decision-making.

The Purpose of Prenatal Check-ups:

Regular prenatal check-ups are a cornerstone of comprehensive prenatal care, offering a systematic approach to monitoring the health and progress of both the expectant mother and the growing fetus. The objectives of these check-ups include:

Assessing Maternal Health:
Monitoring the overall health of the expectant mother, including blood pressure, weight gain, and any existing medical conditions.
Addressing maternal concerns, discomforts, and emotional well-being.

Tracking Fetal Development:
Assessing the growth and development of the fetus through measurements, such as ultrasound scans and fundal height assessments.
Monitoring the baby's heart rate and movements to ensure proper fetal well-being.

Detecting and Managing Complications:
Identifying and addressing any potential complications, such as gestational diabetes, preeclampsia, or infections, in a timely manner.
Developing strategies for managing and minimizing risks to both the mother and the baby.

Providing Education and Support:
Offering information and guidance on nutrition, exercise, and lifestyle choices during pregnancy.
Addressing any questions or concerns the expectant parents may have about childbirth, breastfeeding, and postpartum care.

Establishing a Relationship with Healthcare Providers: Building a trusting and supportive relationship between the expectant parents and their healthcare providers, fostering open communication and shared decision-making.

The Schedule of Prenatal Check-ups:
The frequency of prenatal check-ups varies throughout the course of pregnancy, with more frequent visits in the later stages. A typical schedule for prenatal check-ups includes:

First Trimester (Weeks 4-12):

Initial confirmation of pregnancy with a healthcare provider.
Introduction to prenatal care, including discussions on nutrition, lifestyle, and prenatal vitamins.
Confirmation of gestational age through ultrasound.
Blood tests to assess blood type, Rh factor, and screening for conditions such as anemia.

Second Trimester (Weeks 13-26):

Monthly check-ups in the early second trimester.
Anomaly scan (around 20 weeks) to assess the baby's anatomy and identify potential birth defects.
Glucose tolerance test (around 24-28 weeks) to screen for gestational diabetes.
Monitoring weight gain, blood pressure, and fetal growth.

Third Trimester (Weeks 27-40):

Biweekly check-ups in the early third trimester.
Regular assessments of fetal movements, position, and heart rate.
Monitoring for signs of preeclampsia, including swelling, high blood pressure, and protein in the urine.
Group B streptococcus (GBS) screening around 35-37 weeks.

Weekly Check-ups (Weeks 36-40):

Weekly check-ups in the final weeks of pregnancy to closely monitor maternal and fetal well-being.
Assessing cervical dilation and effacement in preparation for labor.
These are general guidelines, and the frequency of check-ups may vary based on individual circumstances, risk factors, and the recommendations of healthcare providers.

Components of Prenatal Check-ups:

Prenatal check-ups are multifaceted, encompassing various assessments and discussions to comprehensively evaluate and support the health of both the mother and the baby. Key components of these check-ups include:

Physical Examinations:

Regular assessments of maternal vital signs, including blood pressure, heart rate, and respiratory rate.
Monitoring weight gain and addressing any concerns related to edema or swelling.

Fetal Monitoring:
Fetal heart rate monitoring using Doppler ultrasound or electronic fetal monitoring (EFM).
Assessing fetal movements and position through palpation and ultrasound.

Ultrasound Scans:
Scheduled ultrasound scans at different stages of pregnancy to visualize the baby's development and anatomy.
Confirming gestational age, assessing growth, and identifying potential anomalies.

Blood and Urine Tests:
Routine blood tests to assess hemoglobin levels, blood type, Rh factor, and screening for conditions such as gestational diabetes.
Urinalysis to check for signs of infection, protein, or other abnormalities.

Glucose Tolerance Test (GTT):
Conducted around 24-28 weeks to screen for gestational diabetes.
Involves fasting, drinking a glucose solution, and subsequent blood tests to assess glucose levels.

Group B Streptococcus (GBS) Screening:
Performed around 35-37 weeks to identify the presence of GBS bacteria in the genital or rectal area.
Determines the need for antibiotics during labor to prevent transmission to the baby.

Cervical Checks:
In the later stages of pregnancy, cervical checks may be performed to assess dilation and effacement in preparation for labor.

Discussion of Symptoms and Concerns:
An opportunity for the expectant mother to discuss any symptoms, discomforts, or concerns with healthcare providers.
Addressing emotional well-being, stressors, and preparations for labor and postpartum care.

Education and Counseling:
Providing information on nutrition, exercise, and lifestyle choices during pregnancy.
Educating on labor and delivery, breastfeeding, and postpartum care.
Offering support and guidance for a healthy pregnancy journey.

Screening Tests During Pregnancy:
In addition to routine check-ups, various screening tests are conducted during pregnancy to identify potential risks and guide appropriate interventions. These tests include:

First-Trimester Screening:
Nuchal translucency (NT) ultrasound and maternal blood tests to assess the risk of chromosomal abnormalities, including Down syndrome.

Quad Screen or Multiple Marker Screening:
Blood tests performed in the second trimester to assess the risk of neural tube defects and chromosomal abnormalities.

Cell-Free DNA (cfDNA) Testing:
A non-invasive blood test that analyzes fetal DNA in the mother's blood, providing information on chromosomal abnormalities.
Often used as a more accurate screening option, particularly for women at higher risk.
Chorionic Villus Sampling (CVS) and

Amniocentesis:
Diagnostic tests performed if screening tests indicate a higher risk of chromosomal abnormalities.
Involves sampling cells from the placenta (CVS) or amniotic fluid (amniocentesis) for chromosomal analysis.

PHYSICAL CHANGE

BODY CHANGES DURING PREGNANCY

Pregnancy is a miraculous and transformative journey marked by a multitude of physical changes as a woman's body adapts to nurture and support the developing life within. These changes are orchestrated by complex hormonal shifts and the gradual development of the placenta and fetus.

First Trimester (Weeks 1-12):

The first trimester is a critical period marked by the initiation of conception, implantation, and the early stages of fetal development. During these weeks, the body undergoes subtle yet profound changes:

Hormonal Fluctuations:
The body experiences a surge in hormones, particularly human chorionic gonadotropin (hCG) and progesterone. These hormonal changes contribute to common early pregnancy symptoms, including nausea, breast tenderness, and heightened sensitivity to smells.

Breast Changes:
Breasts may become tender and swollen as hormonal shifts prepare the body for breastfeeding.

Darkening of the areolas and the appearance of Montgomery glands, small bumps on the areolas that secrete lubrication for breastfeeding.

Fatigue and Changes in Energy Levels:
Increased progesterone levels can contribute to fatigue as the body redirects energy to support fetal development.
Women may experience changes in sleep patterns, often feeling more tired during the day.

Morning Sickness:
Nausea and vomiting, commonly known as morning sickness, can occur due to hormonal changes.
This symptom varies in intensity and duration among pregnant women.

Frequent Urination:
Increased blood flow to the pelvic area and the growing uterus exert pressure on the bladder.
Frequent urination is a common early pregnancy symptom.

Implantation Bleeding:
Some women may experience light spotting as the fertilized egg implants into the uterine lining.
This is typically brief and lighter than a regular menstrual period.

Uterine Changes:

The uterus begins to expand to accommodate the growing fetus.
Women may feel mild cramping as the uterus undergoes changes to support pregnancy.

Second Trimester (Weeks 13-26):

The second trimester is often referred to as the "honeymoon phase" of pregnancy, marked by a decrease in early pregnancy symptoms and the onset of more visible changes:

Baby Bump Appearance:
The uterus rises above the pelvic bone, and the baby bump becomes more pronounced.
Women often experience a visible "popping" of the belly as the uterus expands.

Skin Changes:
Darkening of the skin, known as chloasma or the "mask of pregnancy," may occur on the face.
Stretch marks may start to appear on the abdomen, breasts, and thighs.

Hair and Nail Changes:
Some women experience thicker, shinier hair due to hormonal influences.
Nails may grow faster and become stronger.

Linea Nigra:

A dark line, called the linea nigra, may appear on the abdomen, running from the pubic bone to the belly button.
This line is caused by increased pigmentation and usually fades after childbirth.

Breathing Changes:
The growing uterus can exert pressure on the diaphragm, leading to shortness of breath.
As the uterus rises, breathing may become easier in the second trimester.

Increased Blood Volume:
Blood volume continues to increase, contributing to a healthy circulatory system for both the mother and the baby.

Baby Movements:
Women may start feeling the baby's movements, known as "quickening."
These movements become more noticeable and regular as the baby grows.

Third Trimester (Weeks 27-40):

The third trimester is characterized by the final stages of pregnancy, with the body preparing for labor and delivery:

Weight Gain:

Weight gain accelerates, with the majority occurring in the third trimester.
This weight gain is attributed to the growing baby, placenta, amniotic fluid, and increased blood volume.

Backache and Joint Pain:
The growing uterus and increased weight can lead to backache and joint pain.
Hormones like relaxin contribute to the relaxation of ligaments, potentially causing discomfort.

Swelling and Edema:
Fluid retention can cause swelling, particularly in the ankles and feet.
Elevation and hydration can help alleviate mild edema.

Braxton Hicks Contractions:
Irregular, painless contractions known as Braxton Hicks contractions may become more noticeable.
These contractions are the body's way of practicing for labor.

Pelvic Pressure:
Pressure on the pelvis increases as the baby descends into the birth canal, preparing for labor.
Women may feel increased pelvic discomfort and the sensation of the baby "dropping."

Increased Vaginal Discharge:
Vaginal discharge may increase as the body produces more mucus to seal the cervix.

This mucus plug protects the uterus from infection.

Shortness of Breath:
As the baby grows and takes up more space, there may
be increased pressure on the diaphragm.
This can lead to shortness of breath and difficulty
breathing deeply.

Physiological Changes Throughout Pregnancy:

Cardiovascular System:
Blood volume increases significantly to support the
needs of the growing fetus.
Heart rate and cardiac output rise to meet the increased
demands on the cardiovascular system.

Respiratory System:
Oxygen consumption and respiratory rate increase,
driven by the needs of the developing fetus.
The diaphragm rises, and tidal volume expands,
contributing to changes in breathing patterns.

Endocrine System:
Hormonal fluctuations, including increased levels of
hCG, progesterone, and estrogen, orchestrate various
physiological changes.
Hormones play a crucial role in maintaining pregnancy,
supporting fetal development, and preparing the body
for labor.

COMMON DISCOMFORTS AND REMEDIES

Pregnancy is a remarkable journey, but it often comes with a range of physical discomforts that arise due to the numerous changes occurring in the expectant mother's body. While these discomforts are typically a natural part of the gestational process, understanding them and exploring effective remedies can significantly improve the overall pregnancy experience.

First Trimester Discomforts:

Morning Sickness:

Description: Nausea and vomiting, commonly referred to as morning sickness, often occur during the first trimester.
Remedies:
Eat small, frequent meals to avoid an empty stomach.
Consume bland, easily digestible foods like crackers or dry toast.
Stay hydrated by sipping ginger or peppermint tea.
Avoid strong odors and consider acupressure wristbands.

Fatigue:

Description: Increased progesterone levels and the energy demands of early pregnancy can lead to pronounced fatigue.
Remedies:

Prioritize rest and take short naps during the day.
Maintain a well-balanced diet with a focus on nutrient-dense foods.
Incorporate light exercises like walking to boost energy levels.

Breast Tenderness:

Description: Hormonal changes cause increased blood flow and sensitivity in the breasts.
Remedies:
Wear a supportive, comfortable bra.
Use warm or cool compresses to alleviate discomfort.
Consider using maternity or sports bras for additional support.

Frequent Urination:

Description: Growing uterus and hormonal changes contribute to increased pressure on the bladder.
Remedies:
Stay hydrated but limit fluids close to bedtime.
Empty the bladder completely when urinating.
Kegel exercises can help strengthen pelvic muscles.

Second Trimester Discomforts:

Backache:

Description: Increased weight and hormonal changes may lead to backache.

Remedies:
Maintain good posture, and use supportive chairs.
Practice prenatal yoga or gentle stretching exercises.
Consider a maternity support belt for added lumbar
support.

Round Ligament Pain:

Description: Sharp, shooting pain due to the stretching
of ligaments supporting the uterus.
Remedies:
Change positions slowly to avoid sudden movements.
Gentle stretching exercises may provide relief.
Warm compresses or a warm bath can alleviate
discomfort.

Leg Cramps:

Description: Painful spasms, often in the calf muscles,
due to changes in circulation and pressure on nerves.
Remedies:
Stay hydrated and maintain a balanced diet with
sufficient calcium and potassium.
Stretching the affected muscle can alleviate cramps.
Massage and warm compresses may provide relief.

Swelling:

Description: Edema or swelling of the ankles and feet
due to increased fluid retention and pressure on blood
vessels.

Remedies:
Elevate legs when sitting or lying down.
Wear comfortable, supportive shoes.
Avoid standing or sitting for extended periods.

Third Trimester Discomforts:

Shortness of Breath:

Description: As the uterus expands, it puts pressure on
the diaphragm, leading to shortness of breath.
Remedies:
Practice deep breathing exercises.
Sleep with extra pillows to elevate the upper body.
Avoid heavy meals, and maintain good posture.

Heartburn and Indigestion:

Description: Hormonal changes relax the esophageal
sphincter, causing stomach acids to rise.
Remedies:
Eat smaller, more frequent meals.
Avoid spicy, acidic, or greasy foods.
Stay upright after meals to aid digestion.

Pelvic Discomfort:

Description: Pressure on the pelvis and pelvic joints may
cause discomfort.
Remedies:
Use a pregnancy pillow for support during sleep.

Pelvic exercises, such as Kegels, may help strengthen muscles.
Warm baths or heat packs can provide relief.

Insomnia:

Description: Difficulty sleeping may arise due to discomfort, hormonal changes, or anxiety.
Remedies:
Establish a relaxing bedtime routine.
Create a comfortable sleep environment.
Practice relaxation techniques, such as meditation or deep breathing.

Throughout Pregnancy:

Constipation:

Description: Slowed digestion and hormonal changes contribute to constipation.
Remedies:
Increase fiber intake through fruits, vegetables, and whole grains.
Stay hydrated by drinking plenty of water.
Gentle exercises, like walking, can stimulate bowel movements.

Varicose Veins:

Description: Enlarged, twisted veins, often in the legs, due to increased pressure on blood vessels.

Remedies:
Elevate legs when resting.
Wear compression stockings.
Avoid standing or sitting for long periods.

Hemorrhoids:

Description: Swollen blood vessels in the rectal area due to increased pressure.
Remedies:
Increase fiber intake and stay hydrated to soften stools.
Avoid straining during bowel movements.
Warm baths and topical treatments can provide relief.

Mood Swings:

Description: Hormonal fluctuations, fatigue, and emotional adjustments can lead to mood swings.
Remedies:
Communicate openly with a partner or support system.
Engage in activities that bring joy and relaxation.
Consider prenatal yoga or mindfulness practices.
General Tips for Managing Discomforts:

Stay Hydrated:
Proper hydration is crucial for overall well-being and can help alleviate some discomforts.

Balanced Diet:

Maintain a well-balanced diet rich in fruits, vegetables, whole grains, and lean proteins to support overall health.

Regular Exercise:
Engage in gentle exercises such as walking, swimming, or prenatal yoga to improve circulation and reduce discomfort.

Support Systems:
Seek support from healthcare providers, friends, and family.
Consider joining prenatal classes or support groups.

Communication:
Communicate openly with healthcare providers about discomforts and concerns.
Share experiences with other expectant mothers for mutual support.

Rest and Relaxation:
Prioritize rest and relaxation to manage fatigue and promote emotional well-being.
Practice relaxation techniques, such as meditation or deep breathing.

Consult Healthcare Providers:
Always consult healthcare providers before trying new remedies or if discomforts persist.

EXERCISE AND STAYING ACTIVE

Pregnancy is a transformative period marked by numerous physical changes, and maintaining a regular exercise routine can contribute significantly to the overall well-being of expectant mothers. Exercise during pregnancy is generally considered safe and beneficial, offering a myriad of advantages for both the mother and the developing baby.

Benefits of Exercise During Pregnancy:

Cardiovascular Health:
Engaging in regular cardiovascular exercise helps maintain a healthy heart and improves circulation, benefiting both the mother and the developing baby.
Enhanced cardiovascular fitness supports the increased demands on the circulatory system during pregnancy.

Gestational Weight Management:
Exercise contributes to healthy weight management during pregnancy, reducing the risk of excessive weight gain.
Maintaining a healthy weight is associated with improved maternal and fetal outcomes.

Muscle Strength and Endurance:
Prenatal exercise, including strength training, helps enhance muscle strength and endurance.

Improved muscular fitness supports the body's changing needs during pregnancy, especially as the uterus and breasts undergo significant growth.

Reduced Discomfort and Fatigue:
Regular exercise can alleviate common discomforts such as backache, leg cramps, and swelling.
Improved muscular strength and flexibility contribute to reduced fatigue and discomfort.

Mood Enhancement:
Exercise stimulates the release of endorphins, promoting a positive mood and reducing stress and anxiety.
Prenatal exercise has been linked to a lower risk of antenatal and postpartum depression.

Improved Sleep Quality:
Physical activity supports better sleep quality during pregnancy.
Establishing a consistent exercise routine can contribute to improved sleep patterns.

Prevention of Gestational Diabetes:
Regular exercise is associated with a reduced risk of gestational diabetes.
Exercise improves insulin sensitivity, helping regulate blood sugar levels.

Enhanced Posture and Balance:

Prenatal exercises that focus on core strength contribute to improved posture and balance.
These benefits are particularly relevant as the body undergoes changes to accommodate the growing uterus.

Preparation for Labor and Delivery:
Physical fitness, including cardiovascular and strength training, may contribute to better endurance during labor.
Improved muscle tone and flexibility support the body's response to the demands of childbirth.

Safe and Recommended Exercises:

Walking:
Walking is a low-impact, accessible exercise suitable for most pregnant women.
It promotes cardiovascular health, boosts mood, and can be easily integrated into daily routines.

Swimming and Water Aerobics:
Water-based exercises are gentle on the joints and provide resistance without impact.
Swimming and water aerobics are effective for cardiovascular fitness and muscle toning.

Prenatal Yoga:
Prenatal yoga focuses on flexibility, relaxation, and breathing techniques.
It helps alleviate tension, improves balance, and enhances overall well-being.

Strength Training:
Moderate strength training with proper form and supervision is generally safe during pregnancy.
Focus on low weights and higher repetitions to build and maintain muscle strength.

Pelvic Floor Exercises (Kegels):
Kegel exercises strengthen the pelvic floor muscles, supporting bladder and bowel control.
Regular practice can be beneficial throughout pregnancy and in postpartum recovery.

Low-Impact Aerobics:
Low-impact aerobics classes designed for pregnant women provide cardiovascular benefits without placing excessive stress on joints.
Ensure the instructor is qualified in prenatal fitness.

Stationary Cycling:
Stationary bikes provide a low-impact cardiovascular workout.
Adjust the bike to a comfortable position and avoid excessive resistance.

Pilates:
Prenatal Pilates focuses on core strength, flexibility, and postural alignment.
Choose classes led by certified instructors with expertise in prenatal fitness.

Safety Considerations and Guidelines:

Consultation with Healthcare Provider:
Before starting or continuing an exercise routine during pregnancy, consult with a healthcare provider.
Discuss any pre-existing medical conditions or pregnancy-related concerns.

Individualized Approach:
Recognize that each pregnancy is unique, and exercise recommendations should be tailored to individual circumstances.
Adjust activities based on fitness level, medical history, and any complications.

Hydration and Temperature Regulation:
Stay well-hydrated, especially during warmer weather.
Avoid overheating, and choose cooler times of the day for outdoor activities.

Listen to Your Body:
Pay attention to how your body responds to exercise.
Modify or stop any activity that causes discomfort, pain, dizziness, or shortness of breath.

Avoid High-Risk Activities:
Refrain from activities with a high risk of falling, abdominal trauma, or excessive joint stress.
Examples include contact sports, high-impact activities, and exercises with a risk of falling.

Pelvic Floor Awareness:
Be mindful of pelvic floor health, especially when performing exercises that involve impact or increased intra-abdominal pressure.
Modify exercises to reduce strain on the pelvic floor.

Appropriate Clothing and Footwear:
Wear comfortable, breathable clothing that accommodates the growing belly.
Choose supportive footwear to prevent foot and ankle discomfort.

Posture Awareness:
Maintain good posture during exercises to reduce strain on the back and spine.
Focus on a neutral spine position and avoid activities that compromise postural alignment.

Modify as Needed:
As pregnancy progresses, modifications may be necessary.
Modify exercises to accommodate the changing center of gravity, balance, and joint laxity.

Postpartum Exercise Transition:
After childbirth, gradually reintroduce exercise based on postpartum recovery.
Resume activities based on individual readiness and healthcare provider guidance.

EMOTIONAL WELL–BEING

HORMONAL CHANGES AND MOOD SWINGS

Pregnancy is a remarkable journey marked not only by physical transformations but also by significant hormonal fluctuations that profoundly impact a woman's emotional well-being. Hormones play a crucial role in orchestrating the complex processes required for the development and sustenance of the growing fetus.

Hormonal Changes Throughout Pregnancy:

First Trimester (Weeks 1-12):

Human Chorionic Gonadotropin (hCG):

Role: Produced by cells in the developing placenta, hCG is crucial for maintaining the corpus luteum, which in turn produces progesterone during early pregnancy.
Impact on Mood: Elevated hCG levels can contribute to heightened emotions and may be linked to early pregnancy symptoms like nausea and mood swings.

Progesterone:

Role: Produced by the corpus luteum in the early stages and later by the placenta, progesterone supports the uterine lining for implantation and helps prevent premature contractions.

Impact on Mood: Increased progesterone levels can lead to drowsiness and, in some cases, mood swings. It acts as a relaxant, affecting the central nervous system.

Estrogen:

Role: Estrogen levels rise significantly during early pregnancy, promoting the growth of the uterus and maintaining the uterine lining.
Impact on Mood: Elevated estrogen can contribute to changes in mood, including increased sensitivity and emotional responsiveness.

Second Trimester (Weeks 13-26):

Progesterone and Estrogen:

Role: Progesterone continues to rise, supporting the uterine environment. Estrogen peaks during the second trimester, influencing fetal development.
Impact on Mood: While mood swings may stabilize for some women, hormonal changes persist, affecting emotions and overall well-being.

Third Trimester (Weeks 27-40):

Oxytocin:

Role: Often referred to as the "love hormone," oxytocin plays a key role in uterine contractions during labor and breastfeeding postpartum.

Impact on Mood: Elevated oxytocin levels may enhance feelings of bonding and attachment, but the anticipation of labor and changes in sleep patterns can contribute to mood fluctuations.

Prolactin:

Role: Released in increasing amounts to prepare the body for breastfeeding.
Impact on Mood: Elevated prolactin levels may be associated with emotional changes, especially as the body prepares for the upcoming demands of breastfeeding.

Hormones and Emotional Well-being:

Hormonal Fluctuations and Emotional Rollercoaster:
The dynamic interplay of hCG, progesterone, estrogen, oxytocin, and prolactin creates a hormonal symphony during pregnancy.
The surge and ebb of these hormones can contribute to mood swings, ranging from elation and joy to moments of heightened sensitivity and tearfulness.

Impact on Stress Response:
Hormones such as cortisol, often associated with stress, can be influenced by the intricate hormonal milieu during pregnancy.
Stress response may vary, impacting how women cope with challenges and emotional stressors.

Individual Variations:
Hormonal responses are highly individual, and genetic, environmental, and lifestyle factors can influence how hormones interact with the brain and the central nervous system.
Expectant mothers may experience varying degrees of mood swings based on their unique hormonal profiles.

Common Mood Swings and Emotional Challenges:

Joy and Elation:

Cause: Hormonal surges, especially oxytocin, can contribute to feelings of joy, contentment, and anticipation.
Impact: Many expectant mothers experience moments of profound happiness and excitement during pregnancy.

Sensitivity and Irritability:

Cause: Hormonal fluctuations, particularly estrogen, can heighten emotional sensitivity.
Impact: Women may find themselves more emotionally reactive or prone to irritability, often in response to stimuli that wouldn't typically trigger such reactions.

Anxiety and Fears:

Cause: The anticipation of labor, changes in lifestyle, and the responsibility of impending motherhood can contribute to anxiety.
Impact: Expectant mothers may grapple with fears related to childbirth, parenting, or concerns about the health of the baby.

Mood Lability:

Cause: Fluctuations in hormones, combined with the physical and emotional demands of pregnancy, can lead to mood lability.
Impact: Rapid shifts in mood, from happiness to sadness or vice versa, are common and often attributed to hormonal changes.

Depressive Symptoms:

Cause: Hormonal imbalances, genetic predispositions, or environmental stressors can contribute to depressive symptoms during pregnancy.
Impact: Some women may experience persistent feelings of sadness, hopelessness, or changes in appetite and sleep patterns.

Coping with Body Image Changes:

Cause: Physical changes, including weight gain and alterations in skin appearance, can impact body image.

Impact: Expectant mothers may grapple with body image concerns, leading to shifts in self-esteem and mood.

Coping Strategies for Mood Swings:

Open Communication:
Openly discuss feelings and concerns with a partner, friends, or healthcare providers.
Establishing a support system can provide a safe space for expressing emotions.

Mindfulness and Relaxation Techniques:
Practice mindfulness, meditation, or deep-breathing exercises to manage stress.
Relaxation techniques can help create a sense of calm amidst emotional fluctuations.

Regular Exercise:
Engage in prenatal exercise to release endorphins and promote emotional well-being.
Activities like yoga or swimming can be particularly beneficial.

Healthy Lifestyle Choices:
Prioritize a balanced diet, stay hydrated, and ensure adequate sleep.
Healthy lifestyle choices contribute to overall well-being and can positively impact mood.

Seek Professional Support:

Consult with mental health professionals if mood swings become overwhelming or depressive symptoms persist. Therapeutic interventions can provide valuable coping strategies.

Educate and Prepare:
Attend prenatal classes to gain knowledge about the birthing process and postpartum expectations.
Education and preparation can alleviate anxiety and fears.

Connect with Other Expectant Mothers:
Join support groups or prenatal classes to connect with other women experiencing similar emotions.
Sharing experiences and advice can foster a sense of community.

Journaling:
Maintain a journal to express thoughts and feelings.
Journaling provides an outlet for self-reflection and emotional processing.

COPING WITH STRESS AND ANXIETY

Stress and anxiety are inevitable aspects of life, but when left unmanaged, they can take a toll on mental and physical well-being. This comprehensive guide explores the intricacies of stress and anxiety, their impact on overall health, and provides an extensive array of coping strategies to foster resilience and maintain a balanced life.

Understanding Stress and Anxiety:

Differentiating Between Stress and Anxiety:

Stress: A response to a specific situation or event, often perceived as a threat or challenge. It is a natural and, in some cases, beneficial reaction.
Anxiety: A more persistent and generalized emotional state characterized by excessive worry, fear, or apprehension. It can be disproportionate to the actual threat.

Physical and Psychological Impact:
Both stress and anxiety can manifest physically through symptoms such as increased heart rate, muscle tension, and digestive issues.
On a psychological level, they can lead to irritability, difficulty concentrating, and disrupted sleep patterns.

Impact on Overall Health:
Chronic stress and anxiety have been linked to various health issues, including cardiovascular problems, weakened immune function, and mental health disorders.
Understanding the interconnectedness of mind and body is crucial for developing effective coping mechanisms.

Root Causes of Stress and Anxiety:

Work-Related Stress:

Causes: High workload, tight deadlines, interpersonal conflicts, and job insecurity.
Coping Strategies: Time management, setting realistic goals, and seeking support from colleagues or supervisors.

Relationship Stress:

Causes: Conflicts, communication breakdowns, or major life changes within relationships.
Coping Strategies: Open communication, couples counseling, and setting healthy boundaries.

Financial Stress:

Causes: Job loss, debt, or financial instability.
Coping Strategies: Budgeting, financial planning, and seeking professional advice when needed.

Health-Related Stress:

Causes: Chronic illnesses, sudden health crises, or concerns about one's health.
Coping Strategies: Regular health check-ups, adopting a healthy lifestyle, and seeking emotional support.

Uncertainty and Change:

Causes: Life transitions, uncertainty about the future, or fear of the unknown.
Coping Strategies: Embracing change, cultivating adaptability, and focusing on what can be controlled.

Coping Strategies for Stress and Anxiety:

Mindfulness and Meditation:

Techniques: Mindfulness meditation, deep-breathing exercises, and progressive muscle relaxation.
Benefits: Enhances present-moment awareness, reduces stress hormones, and promotes overall relaxation.

Regular Exercise:

Types: Aerobic exercises, yoga, and strength training.
Benefits: Releases endorphins, improves mood, and provides a healthy outlet for stress.

Healthy Lifestyle Choices:

Components: Balanced diet, adequate sleep, and regular physical activity.
Benefits: Supports overall well-being, boosts energy levels, and strengthens the body's resilience to stress.

Time Management:

Strategies: Prioritizing tasks, breaking larger goals into smaller steps, and setting realistic deadlines.

Benefits: Reduces feelings of overwhelm, enhances productivity, and creates a sense of accomplishment.

Social Connections:

Activities: Spending time with loved ones, joining social groups, and maintaining a support network.
Benefits: Provides emotional support, fosters a sense of belonging, and helps in perspective-sharing.

Therapeutic Approaches:

Options: Cognitive-Behavioral Therapy (CBT), mindfulness-based therapies, and talk therapy.
Benefits: Offers tools for managing thoughts and emotions, explores coping mechanisms, and provides a supportive space.

Journaling:

Techniques: Reflective journaling, gratitude journaling, or expressive writing.
Benefits: Facilitates self-reflection, clarifies thoughts and emotions, and serves as a therapeutic outlet.

Hobbies and Creative Outlets:

Activities: Art, music, writing, or any creative pursuit.
Benefits: Acts as a form of self-expression, promotes relaxation, and offers a break from stressors.

Setting Boundaries:

Strategies: Clearly communicating limits, learning to say 'no,' and prioritizing self-care.
Benefits: Prevents burnout, fosters healthy relationships, and protects mental well-being.

Mind-Body Techniques:

Practices: Tai Chi, Qigong, and biofeedback.
Benefits: Integrates mental and physical aspects, enhances relaxation, and reduces stress.

Counseling and Support Groups:

Resources: Professional counselors, therapists, or peer support groups.
Benefits: Offers a safe space for expressing feelings, gaining insights, and receiving guidance.

Long-Term Stress Management:

Developing Resilience:

Skills: Problem-solving, adaptability, and optimism.
Benefits: Enhances the ability to bounce back from challenges and navigate stress more effectively.

Mindset Shifts:

Approaches: Embracing a growth mindset, cultivating self-compassion, and reframing negative thoughts.
Benefits: Encourages a positive outlook, reduces self-criticism, and fosters emotional well-being.

Continual Learning:

Areas: Stress management techniques, emotional intelligence, and effective communication.
Benefits: Empowers individuals to proactively address stressors and build a toolkit for ongoing resilience.

Seeking Professional Help:

Recognizing When to Seek Help:

Indicators: Persistent anxiety, overwhelming stress, or interference with daily functioning.
Action: Consulting mental health professionals for assessment and tailored interventions.

Therapeutic Interventions:

Options: Psychotherapy, medication, or a combination of both.
Benefits: Provides specialized support, addresses underlying issues, and offers personalized coping strategies.

Coping with stress and anxiety is a dynamic and ongoing process that requires a multifaceted approach. By understanding the root causes, implementing effective coping strategies, and fostering long-term resilience, individuals can navigate life's challenges with greater ease. The journey towards balanced mental health involves self-discovery, continual learning, and a commitment to prioritizing well-being in the face of life's inevitable stressors.

PARTNER AND FAMILY SUPPORT

The journey of life is often made more meaningful and manageable through the support of loved ones. When it comes to facing challenges, navigating transitions, or celebrating successes, having a strong support system, particularly from a partner and family, can significantly impact overall well-being.

The Importance of Partner and Family Support:

Emotional Resilience:

Role: Partners and family members serve as pillars of emotional support, providing a safe space to express feelings and vulnerabilities.
Impact: Emotional resilience is strengthened when individuals feel understood, valued, and supported in their journey.

Shared Responsibilities:

Role: Partner and family support helps distribute responsibilities, creating a more balanced and manageable life.
Impact: Shared duties lead to reduced stress, allowing individuals to focus on personal and collective growth.

Celebrating Successes:

Role: A supportive network actively participates in celebrating achievements and milestones.
Impact: Shared joy enhances the sense of accomplishment and reinforces a positive environment.

Navigating Challenges:

Role: Partners and family provide a collective strength to face challenges, offering diverse perspectives and solutions.
Impact: Collective problem-solving fosters resilience and minimizes the impact of life's difficulties.

Healthy Communication:

Role: Open and honest communication within a family unit builds trust and strengthens relationships.
Impact: Effective communication is the foundation of healthy relationships, fostering understanding and connection.

Partner Support:

Navigating Life Transitions:

Scenarios: Marriage, parenthood, career changes, or relocation.
Supportive Actions: Listening, expressing empathy, and actively participating in decision-making.

Balancing Responsibilities:

Scenarios: Juggling work, household duties, and personal goals.
Supportive Actions: Equitably dividing tasks, acknowledging each other's contributions, and providing mutual encouragement.

Emotional Support:

Scenarios: Coping with stress, facing challenges, or dealing with personal issues.
Supportive Actions: Offering a listening ear, expressing empathy, and providing reassurance.

Quality Time:

Scenarios: Spending meaningful time together.
Supportive Actions: Planning and prioritizing quality time, engaging in shared activities, and fostering a sense of connection.

Individual Growth:

Scenarios: Pursuing personal goals or self-improvement.
Supportive Actions: Encouraging and supporting individual aspirations, providing constructive feedback, and celebrating personal achievements.

Family Support:

Parental Support:

Scenarios: Parenting challenges, child-rearing decisions, or seeking advice.
Supportive Actions: Sharing responsibilities, offering guidance, and collaborating on parenting decisions.

Sibling Dynamics:

Scenarios: Navigating relationships among siblings.
Supportive Actions: Encouraging positive interactions, mediating conflicts, and fostering a sense of camaraderie.

Extended Family Support:

Scenarios: Dealing with broader family dynamics or seeking assistance.
Supportive Actions: Building connections with extended family members, offering help when needed, and creating a sense of belonging.

Multigenerational Harmony:

Scenarios: Bridging generation gaps and fostering understanding.
Supportive Actions: Encouraging intergenerational relationships, promoting open communication, and respecting diverse perspectives.

Crisis and Trauma:

Scenarios: Coping with family crises or traumatic events.
Supportive Actions: Coming together as a unit, seeking professional help when necessary, and providing emotional support.

Strategies for Fostering Partner and Family Support:

Effective Communication:

Components: Active listening, expressing feelings, and maintaining open dialogue.
Benefits: Enhances understanding, prevents misunderstandings, and promotes a supportive environment.

Quality Time Together:

Activities: Family dinners, outings, and shared hobbies.
Benefits: Strengthens bonds, fosters positive memories, and promotes a sense of togetherness.

Setting Realistic Expectations:

Components: Clear communication about roles, responsibilities, and expectations.
Benefits: Minimizes potential conflicts, fosters a sense of fairness, and encourages collaboration.

Flexibility and Adaptability:

Approach: Embracing change and navigating uncertainties together.
Benefits: Builds resilience, promotes problem-solving, and strengthens the ability to adapt.

Conflict Resolution Skills:

Skills: Active listening, compromise, and finding common ground.
Benefits: Resolves conflicts constructively, strengthens relationships, and maintains a positive family dynamic.

Individual Self-Care:

Encouragement: Promoting self-care practices for each family member.
Benefits: Fosters overall well-being, prevents burnout, and supports a healthier family environment.

Celebrating Achievements:

Actions: Acknowledging and celebrating individual and collective successes.

Benefits: Reinforces a positive environment, boosts morale, and strengthens the sense of accomplishment.

Encouraging Autonomy:

Approach: Supporting individual pursuits and goals.
Benefits: Fosters personal growth, builds confidence, and enriches family dynamics.

Seeking Professional Help:

Indications: Persistent conflicts, challenges, or crises.
Benefits: Professional guidance provides tools for overcoming difficulties, fostering healthier relationships, and enhancing overall family well-being.

The Impact on Different Life Stages:

Early Relationships:

Focus: Establishing a foundation of trust and understanding.
Supportive Actions: Building communication skills, learning about each other's values, and navigating the initial stages of commitment.

Parenthood:

Focus: Navigating the challenges and joys of raising children.

Supportive Actions: Collaborating on parenting decisions, sharing responsibilities, and fostering a united front.

Empty Nest:

Focus: Adjusting to changes after children leave home. Supportive Actions: Rediscovering shared interests, maintaining communication, and supporting each other in new endeavors.

Aging Together:

Focus: Navigating the aging process as a couple or family.
Supportive Actions: Prioritizing health and well-being, addressing challenges together, and ensuring ongoing emotional support.

Partner and family support form the cornerstone of a fulfilling and resilient life. By understanding the importance of these relationships, implementing effective strategies for support, and fostering healthy dynamics, individuals can cultivate an environment that not only navigates challenges but also celebrates shared successes.

PREPARING FOR LABOR AND DELIVERY

CHILDBIRTH EDUCATION CLASSES

Childbirth is a transformative and significant life event, and being well-prepared can make a profound difference in the birthing experience. Childbirth education classes play a crucial role in empowering expectant parents with knowledge, skills, and confidence as they approach labor and delivery.

Understanding Childbirth Education:

Purpose and Goals:

Purpose: Childbirth education classes aim to provide expectant parents with information, tools, and support to make informed decisions about pregnancy, childbirth, and the postpartum period.
Goals: Enhance confidence, promote a positive birthing experience, and foster a sense of empowerment through education.

Timing and Duration:

Timing: Typically taken during the second or third trimester of pregnancy.

Duration: Classes can vary in length, ranging from a one-day intensive course to weekly sessions over several weeks.

Class Formats:

In-Person Classes: Conducted at hospitals, birthing centers, or community centers with a certified childbirth educator.
Online Classes: Offer flexibility and accessibility, allowing parents to participate from the comfort of their homes.

Key Components of Childbirth Education Classes:

Anatomy and Physiology of Pregnancy:

Topics Covered: Changes in the body during pregnancy, fetal development, and the role of the placenta.
Purpose: Understanding the physiological aspects of pregnancy lays the foundation for informed decision-making.

Stages of Labor and Delivery:

Topics Covered: Early labor, active labor, transition, and the pushing stage.
Purpose: Familiarizing parents with the stages of labor helps manage expectations and prepares them for what to expect during each phase.

Pain Management Techniques:

Topics Covered: Breathing exercises, relaxation techniques, positioning, and pain relief options.
Purpose: Equipping parents with a range of coping strategies to manage discomfort and pain during labor.

Medical Interventions:

Topics Covered: Inductions, epidurals, cesarean sections, and other medical interventions.
Purpose: Providing information on common medical interventions allows parents to make informed choices and understand potential implications.

Breastfeeding Education:

Topics Covered: Breastfeeding basics, latching, milk supply, and common challenges.
Purpose: Supporting parents in establishing a positive breastfeeding relationship with their newborns.

Postpartum Care and Recovery:

Topics Covered: Physical and emotional recovery after childbirth, postpartum self-care, and adjusting to life with a newborn.
Purpose: Preparing parents for the postpartum period and helping them recognize and address common challenges.

Newborn Care:

Topics Covered: Diapering, feeding, sleep patterns, and basic newborn care.
Purpose: Offering practical skills and knowledge to build parents' confidence in caring for their newborn.

Informed Decision-Making:

Topics Covered: Understanding the importance of informed consent, asking questions, and advocating for one's preferences.
Purpose: Empowering parents to actively participate in decision-making during childbirth and advocate for their birth preferences.

Emotional and Psychosocial Support:

Topics Covered: Recognizing emotions, communicating with birthing partners, and seeking support.
Purpose: Addressing the emotional aspects of childbirth and providing tools for effective communication and support.

Benefits of Childbirth Education Classes:

Empowerment:

Impact: Parents feel more empowered with knowledge, leading to increased confidence in their ability to navigate the birthing process.

Reduced Anxiety and Fear:

Impact: Education about the birthing process helps alleviate anxiety and fear by demystifying the unknown and providing a sense of control.

Partner Involvement:

Impact: Partners become active participants in the birthing experience, offering support and understanding their role during labor and delivery.

Improved Communication:

Impact: Parents learn effective communication skills, enhancing their ability to express preferences, concerns, and needs to healthcare providers.

Informed Decision-Making:

Impact: Parents are equipped to make informed decisions about their birthing experience, ensuring their preferences align with the available options.

Postpartum Preparation:

Impact: Education about postpartum care and recovery helps parents anticipate and navigate challenges in the early weeks after childbirth.

Building a Support Network:

Impact: Classes provide an opportunity for expectant parents to connect with each other, fostering a supportive community.

Breastfeeding Success:

Impact: Breastfeeding education increases the likelihood of successful breastfeeding initiation and duration.

HOSPITAL BAG ESSENTIALS

Preparing for the arrival of a new family member is an exciting and monumental task. One essential aspect of this preparation is putting together a hospital bag that includes everything you might need during your stay for labor, delivery, and the initial postpartum period.

Planning and Timing:

When to Pack:

Third Trimester: It's advisable to have your hospital bag ready by the beginning of the third trimester to ensure you're prepared for any unexpected early arrivals.

Check Hospital Policies:

Guidelines: Some hospitals may provide a checklist or guidelines for what to pack, so check with your healthcare provider or the hospital where you plan to give birth.

Essential Documents:

Identification and Insurance:

Driver's License/ID: Ensure you have a form of identification.
Insurance Information: Carry your insurance card and any necessary pre-authorization documents.

Birth Plan:

Printed Copy: Have a printed copy of your birth plan, if you have one, to discuss with your healthcare team.

Hospital Registration Forms:

Completed Forms: If there are any pre-registration forms, ensure they are completed and packed.

Medical Records:

Prenatal Records: Copies of your prenatal records or any relevant medical information.

Clothing for Labor and Delivery:

Comfortable Labor Attire:

Loose, Comfortable Outfit: Pack a loose and comfortable outfit for labor, like a loose-fitting nightgown or a comfortable robe.

Warm Socks:

Non-Slip: Choose non-slip socks with grips to keep your feet warm and provide traction.

Supportive Bra:

Sports Bra or Nursing Bra: A supportive bra can be essential during labor.

Comfortable Underwear:

High-Waisted and Disposable: High-waisted, disposable underwear is comfortable and convenient.

Hair Ties or Headbands:

Keep Hair Tied Back: Having your hair out of your face can be helpful during labor.

Postpartum Clothing:

Comfortable Pajamas or Nightgowns:

Front-Opening for Breastfeeding: Front-opening pajamas or nightgowns make breastfeeding easier.

Robe:

Comfort and Modesty: A soft robe provides comfort and modesty when receiving visitors or walking around the hospital.

Slippers or Comfortable Shoes:

Easy to Slip On: Comfortable footwear for walking around the hospital.

Nursing Bras and Breast Pads:

Supportive Bras: Nursing bras and breast pads for comfort and leakage.

Comfortable Underwear:

High-Waisted and Breathable: High-waisted, breathable underwear is essential for postpartum recovery.

Toiletries:

Toothbrush and Toothpaste:

Travel Size: Travel-sized toothbrush and toothpaste for maintaining oral hygiene.

Shampoo and Conditioner:

Travel Size: Compact sizes of your preferred shampoo and conditioner.

Body Wash or Soap:

Gentle and Fragrance-Free: Opt for a gentle, fragrance-free soap.

Hairbrush or Comb:

Detangling: A brush or comb for managing your hair.

Face Wash:

Mild and Hypoallergenic: A mild and hypoallergenic face wash.

Deodorant:

Unscented: Choose an unscented deodorant.

Lip Balm:

Hydrating: Hospitals can be dry, so a hydrating lip balm is useful.

Glasses or Contact Lenses:

Lens Case and Solution: If you wear contacts, bring a case and solution.

Comfort Items:

Pillow from Home:

Comfort: A familiar pillow can provide comfort during your hospital stay.

Blanket:

Warmth and Familiarity: A cozy blanket or throw from home.

Comfortable Socks or Slippers:

Warmth and Comfort: Additional warm socks or comfortable slippers for walking around.

Eye Mask and Earplugs:

Sleep Aid: Useful for creating a restful environment.

Aromatherapy:

Essential Oils or Scented Sachets: If allowed, bring calming scents for relaxation.

Electronics and Entertainment:

Phone and Charger:

Fully Charged: Keep your phone charged for communication and entertainment.

Camera or Video Camera:

Capture Memories: If you prefer, a camera for capturing special moments.

Tablet or E-Reader:

Entertainment: Loaded with e-books, movies, or games for downtime.

Headphones:

Privacy: Provide a bit of privacy and block out noise.

Snacks and Hydration:

Healthy Snacks:

Nutritious Options: Pack snacks like nuts, granola bars, or dried fruit for energy.

Reusable Water Bottle:

Hydration: Staying hydrated during labor is important, so bring a reusable water bottle.

For the Baby:

Going-Home Outfit:

Weather-Appropriate: An outfit for your baby to wear when leaving the hospital.

Blanket or Swaddle:

Comfort: A soft blanket or swaddle for your baby.
Newborn Diapers and Wipes:

Hospital May Provide: Some hospitals provide these, but it's good to have a backup.

Car Seat:

Installed Correctly: Ensure your car seat is correctly installed for the journey home.

Miscellaneous Items:

Important Contacts:

Contact List: Keep a list of important contacts, including family members, friends, and your healthcare provider.

Notebook and Pen:

Recording Thoughts: Useful for jotting down thoughts, questions, or memories.

Insurance Information:

Emergency: A copy of your insurance information for any unexpected situations.

Snack for the Support Person:

Energy: A snack for your partner or support person during labor.

Folder for Paperwork:

Organization: Keep all important paperwork and documents in a folder for easy access.

NEWBORN CARE

BASICS OF BABY CARE

Bringing a new baby into the world is a joyous and transformative experience, but it also comes with a multitude of new responsibilities and challenges. Understanding the basics of baby care is crucial for new parents, helping them navigate the early days and weeks with confidence.

Feeding Your Baby:

Breastfeeding:

Positioning and Latching: Ensure a comfortable and proper latch for effective breastfeeding.
Frequency: Newborns typically feed every 2-3 hours, but feeding on demand is essential.
Pumping and Storing Milk: If expressing breast milk, learn proper pumping techniques and safe storage practices.

Formula Feeding:

Choosing Formula: Select a formula that meets your baby's nutritional needs.
Bottle Feeding Techniques: Learn the proper way to hold and feed your baby with a bottle.

Introducing Solid Foods:

Timing: Begin introducing solids around 6 months, following your baby's cues.
Single-Ingredient Foods: Start with single-ingredient foods to monitor for allergies.
Gradual Introduction: Introduce new foods one at a time and wait a few days before adding another.

Hydration:

Breast Milk or Formula: Until the introduction of solids, breast milk or formula provides sufficient hydration.
Introducing Water: Once solids are introduced, offer small sips of water.

Diapering and Hygiene:

Diaper Changing:

Frequency: Newborns may need changing every 2-3 hours, or whenever they are wet or soiled.
Proper Technique: Ensure a clean and safe diaper changing area.
Diaper Rash Prevention: Use diaper cream and change diapers promptly to prevent diaper rash.

Bathing:

Frequency: 2-3 times a day is usually sufficient for newborns.

Gentle Cleansing Products: Use mild, fragrance-free soap and shampoo for sensitive baby skin.
Temperature and Safety: Check water temperature and never leave the baby unattended during a bath.

Umbilical Cord Care:

Gentle Cleaning: Clean the area with a cotton swab and rubbing alcohol until the stump falls off.
Avoid Submersion: Avoid submerging the baby in water until the stump has completely healed.

Nail Care:

Regular Trimming: Trim baby's nails regularly to prevent scratching.
Safety First: Use baby-safe nail clippers and ensure good lighting.

Sleeping:

Safe Sleep Environment:

Back to Sleep: Always place your baby on their back to sleep.
Firm Mattress: Use a firm mattress with a fitted sheet.
No Loose Bedding: Avoid blankets, pillows, and soft toys in the crib to reduce the risk of SIDS.

Sleep Routine:

Consistent Schedule: Establish a consistent sleep routine to help your baby differentiate between day and night.
Creating a Calm Environment: Dim the lights and engage in calming activities before bedtime.

Understanding Newborn Sleep Patterns:

Frequent Waking: Newborns wake frequently for feeding and diaper changes.
Napping: Encourage napping during the day to ensure adequate rest.

Health and Wellness:

Well-Baby Checkups:

Regular Appointments: Schedule regular checkups with your pediatrician to monitor growth and development.
Vaccinations: Follow the recommended vaccination schedule to protect against preventable diseases.

Signs of Illness:

Fever: Learn how to measure and respond to a baby's fever.
Seeking Medical Attention: Recognize signs of illness and know when to contact your healthcare provider.

Cord Blood Banking:

Information Gathering: Consider gathering information on cord blood banking and discuss the option with your healthcare provider.

Developmental Milestones:

Tracking Progress: Understand age-appropriate milestones for physical, cognitive, and social development.
Encouraging Interaction: Engage in activities that promote sensory and motor development.

Tummy Time:

Regular Sessions: Incorporate daily tummy time to strengthen neck and upper body muscles.
Supervised: Always supervise tummy time to ensure the baby's safety.

Comfort and Soothing Techniques:

Swaddling:

Technique: Learn the proper way to swaddle, providing comfort and security.
Safe Sleep Practices: Swaddle for sleep following safe sleep guidelines.

Pacifiers:

Soothing Tool: Offer a pacifier for comfort and to satisfy the baby's natural sucking reflex.
Weaning: Begin weaning off pacifier use when appropriate.

Cuddling and Holding:

Bonding: Frequent cuddling and holding promote bonding between parents and the baby.
Kangaroo Care: Practice skin-to-skin contact for added bonding benefits.

Music and White Noise:

Calming Sounds: Use soft music or white noise machines to create a soothing environment.
Establishing Sleep Cues: Consistent sounds can become sleep cues for the baby.

Baby Gear and Essentials:

Diapers and Wipes:

Stocking Up: Ensure an ample supply of diapers and wipes.
Diaper Bag: Keep a well-packed diaper bag for outings.

Clothing:

Seasonal Wardrobe: Dress the baby appropriately for the weather.

Comfortable Sleepwear: Choose comfortable sleepwear for bedtime.

Baby Carrier or Sling:

Hands-Free Comfort: Use a baby carrier or sling for hands-free carrying.
Proper Positioning: Ensure proper positioning to support the baby's developing spine.

Stroller:

Choosing the Right Stroller: Select a stroller that suits your lifestyle and provides comfort for the baby.
Safety Considerations: Ensure the stroller meets safety standards.

Car Seat:

Proper Installation: Install the car seat correctly before the baby's arrival.
Periodic Checks: Regularly check the car seat for proper fit and adjustments.

Baby Monitor:

Audio or Video: Choose a baby monitor with audio and/or video capabilities.
Monitoring Sleep: Use the monitor to keep an eye on the baby during sleep.

Parental Self-Care:

Rest and Nutrition:

Prioritizing Rest: Nap when the baby naps to ensure sufficient rest.
Balanced Diet: Maintain a balanced diet to support your energy levels.

BREASTFEEDING OR FORMULA FEEDING

The decision between breastfeeding and formula feeding is one of the first major choices new parents face. Both options come with their unique benefits and challenges, and the decision often involves considering various factors such as lifestyle, health considerations, and personal preferences.

Breastfeeding:

Benefits for the Baby:

Nutritional Superiority: Breast milk is a complete and easily digestible source of nutrition for infants.
Immune System Support: Provides antibodies that help protect the baby from infections and illnesses.
Optimal Brain Development: Contains essential fatty acids crucial for brain development.

Benefits for the Mother:

Bonding: Enhances the emotional connection between mother and baby.
Postpartum Recovery: Aids in uterine contraction, helping the mother's body recover after childbirth.
Reduced Risk of Certain Diseases: Linked to a decreased risk of breast cancer, ovarian cancer, and postpartum depression.

Convenience:

Always Available: Breast milk is readily available at the right temperature, eliminating the need for preparation.
Cost-Free: Breastfeeding is cost-free compared to the ongoing expense of formula.

Environmental Impact:

Eco-Friendly: Producing breast milk has a significantly lower environmental impact than formula production and packaging.

Customized Nutrition:

Adapts to Baby's Needs: Breast milk composition changes to meet the evolving nutritional needs of the baby.

Health Benefits for the Baby:

Reduced Risk of Infections: Breastfed babies are less likely to develop respiratory and gastrointestinal infections.
Lowered Risk of Allergies: Linked to a decreased risk of allergies and eczema.
Reduced Risk of Sudden Infant Death Syndrome (SIDS): Breastfeeding is associated with a lower risk of SIDS.

Promotion of Healthy Weight:

Reduced Risk of Childhood Obesity: Breastfed babies are less likely to become overweight later in childhood.

Postpartum Weight Loss:

Caloric Expenditure: Burns extra calories, aiding in postpartum weight loss for the mother.

Breastfeeding as Birth Control:

Lactational Amenorrhea Method (LAM): Exclusive breastfeeding can serve as a natural form of birth control during the first six months, though effectiveness varies.

Challenges of Breastfeeding:

Initial Latching and Positioning:

Learning Curve: Some babies and mothers may experience challenges in achieving a proper latch and comfortable positioning.

Sore Nipples: Initial soreness or discomfort as both mother and baby adjust to breastfeeding.

Frequency and Duration:

Demanding Schedule: Breastfed babies often feed more frequently, which can be time-consuming.
Night Feedings: Night feedings may be more frequent compared to formula-fed babies.

Public Perception and Comfort:

Social Stigma: Public breastfeeding may face social stigma or discomfort in certain settings.
Privacy Concerns: Some mothers may feel uncomfortable breastfeeding in public.

Maternal Time and Commitment:

Time-Intensive: Breastfeeding requires a significant time commitment from the mother.
Challenges with Pumping: Working mothers may face challenges with pumping and storing breast milk.

Dietary Limitations for the Mother:

Dietary Impact: Some mothers may feel limited in their dietary choices due to the impact on breast milk.
Alcohol and Medication Considerations: Mothers need to be cautious with alcohol consumption and medication.

Formula Feeding:

Flexibility and Convenience:

Ease of Use: Formula feeding provides flexibility as anyone can participate in feeding the baby.
Convenient for Working Mothers: Allows working mothers to share feeding responsibilities with other caregivers.

Predictable Feeding Schedule:

Regular Intervals: Formula-fed babies may go longer between feedings compared to breastfed babies.
Night Sleep: May have longer stretches of sleep at night compared to breastfed babies.

Nutrient Consistency:

Standardized Nutrition: Formula provides consistent nutrition, making it easier to monitor the baby's intake.
Visibility of Intake: Allows caregivers to precisely measure how much the baby is consuming.

Maternal Freedom:

Freedom of Diet: Mothers have more dietary freedom as their food choices do not impact the composition of formula.

Freedom of Schedule: Easier to plan outings and work schedules without the need for breastfeeding.

Easier to Share Responsibilities:

Equal Participation: Allows other caregivers, including partners, family members, or childcare providers, to take an active role in feeding.
Reduced Maternal Exhaustion: Sharing feeding responsibilities can help prevent maternal exhaustion.

Reduced Physical Demands:

Physical Recovery: Formula feeding may be less physically demanding for some mothers.
Reduced Breast Discomfort: Absence of breastfeeding may alleviate breast-related discomfort.

Challenges of Formula Feeding:

Cost:

Ongoing Expense: Formula feeding incurs ongoing costs for purchasing formula and related accessories.

Lack of Immune Protections:

Reduced Immune Support: Formula-fed babies may not benefit from the immune-boosting properties found in breast milk.

Increased Risk of Infections: Formula-fed babies may be at a slightly higher risk of respiratory and gastrointestinal infections.

Preparation and Cleanliness:

Time-Consuming Preparation: Formula preparation involves more time and cleanliness considerations.
Sterilization Requirements: Sterilization of bottles and nipples is essential to prevent infections.

Environmental Impact:

Carbon Footprint: Formula production and packaging contribute to a larger carbon footprint compared to breastfeeding.

Specific Health Risks for the Baby:

Gastrointestinal Issues: Formula-fed babies may experience more constipation or gastrointestinal discomfort.
Increased Risk of Allergies: Some studies suggest a slightly higher risk of allergies in formula-fed infants.

Combination Feeding (Mixed Feeding):

Definition:

Alternating Breastfeeding and Formula Feeding: Combines both breastfeeding and formula feeding based on the parents' preferences and circumstances.

Flexibility:

Adaptability: Offers flexibility, allowing parents to choose the feeding method based on their daily routines and preferences.
Shared Responsibility: Allows both parents or caregivers to share feeding responsibilities.

Reduced Pressure on the Mother:

Balancing Work and Breastfeeding: Eases the challenges working mothers face in balancing work schedules and breastfeeding.
Maternal Well-Being: Provides a compromise that may reduce maternal stress and pressure.

SLEEP SCHEDULES AND ROUTINES

Quality sleep is crucial for overall health and well-being, and establishing effective sleep schedules and routines plays a pivotal role in ensuring restful and rejuvenating sleep.

Understanding the Science of Sleep:

Sleep Architecture:

Stages of Sleep: Explore the different sleep stages, including REM (Rapid Eye Movement) and non-REM sleep.
Sleep Cycles: Understand the cyclical nature of sleep cycles and their impact on overall sleep quality.

Circadian Rhythms:

Biological Clock: Learn about circadian rhythms and how they regulate the sleep-wake cycle.
Impact of Light: Understand how exposure to light, especially natural sunlight, influences circadian rhythms.

Sleep Needs Across Ages:

Infants and Newborns: Recognize the high sleep requirements for infants, including frequent napping.
Children and Adolescents: Understand the evolving sleep needs of children and the impact of puberty on sleep patterns.
Adults and Seniors: Explore the changes in sleep architecture and duration as people age.

Importance of Healthy Sleep:

Physical Health:

Immune Function: Quality sleep supports a robust immune system.

Growth and Development: Crucial for growth, particularly in children and adolescents.

Mental Health:

Emotional Regulation: Sleep influences emotional resilience and the ability to cope with stress.
Cognitive Function: Essential for cognitive functions such as memory, attention, and problem-solving.

Overall Well-Being:

Mood Regulation: Adequate sleep is linked to better mood regulation and a lower risk of mood disorders.
Metabolic Health: Impacts metabolism, weight regulation, and the risk of metabolic disorders.

Sleep Requirements Across Age Groups:

Infants (0-12 months):

Total Sleep Time: Newborns may sleep up to 16-20 hours a day, with shorter sleep cycles.
Napping: Frequent napping is common, and sleep is often divided into multiple short periods.

Children (1-5 years):

Total Sleep Time: Ranges from 10 to 14 hours, including naps.

Bedtime Routine: Establishing a consistent bedtime routine is crucial.

School-Age Children (6-12 years):

Total Sleep Time: Recommended 9-12 hours of sleep per night.
Consistent Sleep Schedule: Maintaining a consistent sleep schedule, including weekends, is beneficial.

Teenagers (13-18 years):

Total Sleep Time: Recommended 8-10 hours, but biological changes may shift sleep-wake patterns.
Sleep Hygiene: Emphasize the importance of a consistent sleep routine and minimizing screen time before bedtime.

Adults (18-64 years):

Total Sleep Time: Generally 7-9 hours, but individual needs may vary.
Regular Sleep Schedule: Consistency in bedtime and wake-up times is essential.

Seniors (65 years and older):

Total Sleep Time: May experience a shift in sleep architecture, with lighter sleep and more frequent awakenings.

Daytime Napping: Short naps can be beneficial, but excessive daytime sleep may impact nighttime sleep.

Common Sleep Issues:

Insomnia:

Difficulty Falling Asleep: Explore strategies to improve sleep onset.
Interrupted Sleep: Addressing factors contributing to frequent awakenings during the night.

Sleep Apnea:

Breathing Interruptions: Recognize symptoms of sleep apnea and seek medical evaluation if necessary.
Treatment Options: Explore interventions such as continuous positive airway pressure (CPAP) therapy.

Restless Legs Syndrome (RLS):

Uncomfortable Sensations: Understand the symptoms of RLS and consider lifestyle adjustments or medical treatments.

Narcolepsy:

Excessive Daytime Sleepiness: Recognize signs of narcolepsy and consult a healthcare professional for diagnosis and management.

Circadian Rhythm Disorders:

Shift Work Sleep Disorder: Strategies for managing sleep when working irregular hours.
Jet Lag: Tips for mitigating the effects of time zone changes on sleep.

Parasomnias:

Nightmares and Night Terrors: Strategies for managing and reducing the frequency of parasomnias.

Creating Healthy Sleep Routines:

Establishing Consistent Bedtimes:

All Ages: Maintain a regular bedtime, even on weekends.
Bedtime Rituals: Develop calming rituals before bedtime to signal the body that it's time to wind down.

Creating a Relaxing Sleep Environment:

Ideal Room Conditions: Keep the bedroom cool, dark, and quiet.
Comfortable Mattress and Bedding: Invest in a comfortable mattress and pillows.

Limiting Screen Time Before Bed:

All Ages: Minimize exposure to screens at least an hour before bedtime.

Blue Light Filters: Consider using blue light filters on electronic devices.

Encouraging Physical Activity:

All Ages: Promote regular physical activity, but avoid vigorous exercise close to bedtime.

Healthy Eating Habits:

Avoiding Heavy Meals: Discourage large, heavy meals close to bedtime.
Limiting Caffeine and Sugar: Encourage moderation in caffeine and sugar intake, especially in the evening.

Managing Stress:

All Ages: Teach stress management techniques, such as deep breathing or mindfulness.
Bedtime Reflection: Encourage positive thoughts and reflection before bedtime.

Age-Appropriate Sleep Schedules:

Children and Adolescents: Align sleep schedules with school requirements and extracurricular activities.
Adults: Develop sleep schedules that accommodate work demands and personal preferences.

Consistent Wake-Up Times:

All Ages: Maintain a consistent wake-up time, even on weekends.
Morning Sun Exposure: Exposure to natural sunlight in the morning can help regulate circadian rhythms.

Managing Sleep Transitions:

Transitioning from Cribs to Beds:

Gradual Transition: Make the transition gradually, ensuring the child feels comfortable in the new sleeping environment.
Positive Associations: Create positive associations with the new bed.

Adjusting to School Schedules:

Consistent Wake-Up Times: Maintain consistent wake-up times, even during school breaks.
Earlier Bedtime: Gradually adjust bedtime as the school start date approaches.

POSTPARTUM RECOVERY

PHYSICAL RECOVERY FOR MOMS

The postpartum period is a transformative and challenging time for new mothers, both physically and emotionally. Proper physical recovery is essential for the well-being of moms as they adapt to the changes in their bodies after childbirth.

Understanding the Postpartum Body:

Postpartum Healing:

Uterine Contractions: The uterus undergoes contractions, known as afterpains, to return to its pre-pregnancy size.
Lochia Discharge: Postpartum bleeding, called lochia, is normal and can last for several weeks.

Perineal Healing:

Episiotomy or Tears: Care for stitches or tears in the perineal area with proper hygiene and pain management.
Sitz Baths: Warm water baths can aid in perineal healing and reduce discomfort.

Breast Changes:

Engorgement: Manage breast engorgement with proper breastfeeding techniques or expressing milk.
Cracked Nipples: Address issues like cracked nipples promptly for successful breastfeeding.

Abdominal Changes:

Diastasis Recti: Understand abdominal separation and engage in exercises to promote healing.
Postpartum Belly Binding: Evaluate the benefits of postpartum belly binding for some women.

Pelvic Floor Health:

Kegel Exercises: Strengthen pelvic floor muscles with kegel exercises to aid in recovery.
Pelvic Floor Therapy: Consider pelvic floor physical therapy for specific concerns.

Nutrition for Postpartum Recovery:

Hydration:

Importance of Water: Stay adequately hydrated, especially for breastfeeding mothers.
Limiting Caffeine and Sugary Drinks: Be mindful of caffeine and sugary beverages that can affect hydration levels.

Balanced Diet:

Nutrient-Rich Foods: Consume a diet rich in fruits, vegetables, lean proteins, and whole grains.
Iron-Rich Foods: Address postpartum anemia with iron-rich foods or supplements if recommended by a healthcare professional.

Postpartum Superfoods:

Oats, Salmon, and Leafy Greens: Incorporate superfoods that support energy levels, lactation, and overall recovery.

Supplements:

Prenatal Vitamins: Continue taking prenatal vitamins as recommended by a healthcare provider.
Omega-3 Fatty Acids: Omega-3 supplements can support postpartum mental health and breastfeeding.

Meal Preparation and Planning:

Batch Cooking: Prepare and freeze nutritious meals for easy access during busy postpartum days.
Snack Options: Have healthy snacks readily available for quick and convenient nourishment.

Exercise and Physical Activity:

Postpartum Exercise Guidelines:

Consultation with Healthcare Provider: Obtain clearance from a healthcare provider before starting any postpartum exercise routine.
Gradual Progression: Gradually reintroduce exercise, starting with gentle activities like walking.

Pelvic Floor Exercises:

Kegels and Beyond: Incorporate pelvic floor exercises into the postpartum fitness routine.
Yoga and Pilates: Explore yoga or Pilates classes tailored to postpartum recovery.

Cardiovascular Exercise:

Low-Impact Options: Begin with low-impact cardiovascular exercises such as swimming or stationary cycling.
Postpartum Running: Gradually reintroduce running after receiving approval from a healthcare provider.

Strength Training:

Focus on Core Strength: Strengthen the core muscles with postpartum-friendly exercises.
Full-Body Workouts: Incorporate full-body strength training for overall fitness.

Postpartum Fitness Classes:

Specialized Classes: Explore postpartum fitness classes designed for new moms.
Mom and Baby Classes: Attend classes that allow mothers to exercise with their babies.

Rest and Sleep:

Prioritizing Rest:

Quality Over Quantity: Focus on quality sleep, even if the duration is fragmented during the early postpartum period.
Sleep When the Baby Sleeps: Prioritize napping when the baby is asleep to support recovery.

Establishing Sleep Routines:

Consistent Bedtime: Develop a regular bedtime routine to signal the body that it's time to wind down.
Creating a Comfortable Sleep Environment: Make the bedroom conducive to restful sleep.

Napping Strategies:

Strategic Napping: Take short naps strategically to combat fatigue.
Avoiding Long Naps: Minimize long naps during the day to prevent disruptions to nighttime sleep.

Mental Health and Emotional Well-Being:

Addressing Postpartum Blues and Depression:

Seeking Support: Talk to healthcare providers, support groups, or mental health professionals if experiencing symptoms of postpartum blues or depression.
Open Communication: Share feelings and concerns with partners, friends, and family.

Stress Management Techniques:

Mindfulness and Meditation: Incorporate mindfulness and meditation practices to manage stress.
Breathing Exercises: Practice deep breathing exercises for relaxation.

The Role of Support Systems:

Partner Involvement:

Shared Responsibilities: Encourage partners to share responsibilities in childcare and household chores.
Emotional Support: Offer emotional support and open communication.

Family and Friends:

Assistance with Tasks: Welcome help from family and friends with tasks like meal preparation and errands.
Providing Emotional Support: Surround yourself with individuals who offer emotional support during the postpartum period.

Community and Peer Support:

Joining Mom Groups: Participate in local mom groups or online communities to connect with other new mothers.
Sharing Experiences: Share experiences and seek advice from peers who have gone through similar postpartum journeys.

Pelvic Floor Rehabilitation:

Pelvic Floor Physical Therapy:

Consultation with a Specialist: Consider pelvic floor physical therapy for personalized guidance.
Exercises and Techniques: Learn specific exercises and techniques to address pelvic floor concerns.

Incorporating Pelvic Floor Exercises:

Kegels and Beyond: Integrate pelvic floor exercises into daily routines to promote recovery.
Yoga and Pilates: Explore specialized yoga or Pilates classes focusing on pelvic floor health.

EMOTIONAL ADJUSTMENTS

Emotions are an integral part of the human experience, shaping our perceptions, decisions, and overall well-being. Throughout life, individuals encounter a myriad of transitions and challenges that necessitate emotional adjustments.

Understanding Emotions:

Emotional Intelligence:

Definition: Explore the concept of emotional intelligence and its components.
Importance: Understand how emotional intelligence contributes to overall personal and professional success.

Basic Emotions:

Primary Emotions: Examine fundamental emotions like happiness, sadness, anger, fear, surprise, and disgust.
Universal Expressions: Recognize that certain emotional expressions are universally understood across cultures.

Complex Emotions:

Mixed Emotions: Delve into nuanced emotions that arise from the interplay of primary emotions.
Secondary Emotions: Understand the layers of emotions that emerge in response to specific situations.

Emotion Regulation:

Definition: Explore the ability to manage and modulate one's emotional responses.

Strategies: Learn effective strategies for emotion regulation, including mindfulness and cognitive reappraisal.

Emotional Adjustments Across Life Stages:

Childhood and Adolescence:

Identity Formation: Explore emotional adjustments related to the formation of identity during adolescence.
Peer Relationships: Understand the impact of peer relationships on emotional well-being.

Young Adulthood:

Transitions: Navigate emotional adjustments related to leaving home, pursuing education, and establishing independence.
Relationships and Intimacy: Explore the emotional landscape of forming romantic relationships and navigating intimacy.

Adulthood:

Career and Family Dynamics: Understand the emotional complexities of balancing career aspirations and family responsibilities.
Parenting Challenges: Explore the emotional adjustments involved in becoming a parent and raising children.

Midlife:

Identity Reevaluation: Address emotional shifts associated with reevaluating life goals and priorities.
Empty Nest Syndrome: Understand the emotional impact when children leave home.

Later Life:

Retirement and Aging: Explore emotional adjustments related to retirement, aging, and changes in physical health.
Loss and Grief: Understand the emotional challenges associated with loss and bereavement.

Navigating Life Transitions:

Resilience Building:

Definition: Explore the concept of resilience and its role in navigating life's challenges.
Building Resilience: Learn strategies for developing resilience, including fostering social connections and maintaining a positive outlook.

Coping with Change:

Adaptive Coping Strategies: Explore healthy coping mechanisms to deal with unexpected life changes.

Seeking Support: Understand the importance of seeking support from friends, family, or mental health professionals.

Managing Stress:

Identifying Stressors: Recognize common sources of stress in daily life.
Stress Management Techniques: Explore effective stress management techniques, including mindfulness, exercise, and time management.

Adapting to New Environments:

Relocation and Cultural Adjustments: Address the emotional challenges associated with moving to a new place or adapting to a different culture.
Embracing Change: Develop a mindset that embraces change as an opportunity for personal growth.

Cultivating Emotional Well-Being:

Self-Reflection and Awareness:

Mindfulness Practices: Explore mindfulness and meditation as tools for self-reflection and emotional awareness.
Journaling: Develop a habit of journaling to process emotions and gain insights into personal experiences.

Positive Psychology:

Focus on Strengths: Adopt a positive psychology approach by identifying and leveraging personal strengths.
Gratitude Practices: Cultivate gratitude through daily practices to enhance emotional well-being.

Healthy Relationships:

Communication Skills: Develop effective communication skills to foster healthy relationships.
Boundaries: Establish and maintain boundaries to support emotional well-being in relationships.

Embracing Vulnerability:

Brené Brown's Insights: Explore the concept of vulnerability and its role in building authentic connections.
Risk-Taking and Growth: Understand how embracing vulnerability can lead to personal and emotional growth.

Pursuing Passions and Hobbies:

Identifying Interests: Explore and engage in activities that bring joy and fulfillment.
Work-Life Balance: Strive for a healthy balance between personal interests and professional responsibilities.

Physical Health and Exercise:

Mind-Body Connection: Recognize the interconnectedness of physical and emotional health.
Exercise and Mood: Understand the positive impact of regular exercise on mood and emotional well-being.

Mental Health and Professional Support:

Recognizing Mental Health Concerns:

Common Mental Health Conditions: Learn about common mental health conditions, including anxiety and depression.
Reducing Stigma: Address the stigma surrounding mental health issues to encourage seeking help.

Seeking Professional Support:

Therapy and Counseling: Understand the benefits of therapy and counseling in addressing emotional challenges.
Medication and Psychiatry: Explore the role of medication and psychiatric support in managing mental health conditions.

Online Resources and Support Groups:

Accessibility: Utilize online resources and support groups for convenient access to emotional support.
Community Connection: Engage with online communities that provide a sense of connection and shared experiences.

Family Dynamics and Emotional Adjustments:

Parenting Challenges:

Balancing Responsibilities: Address the emotional adjustments involved in balancing parenting responsibilities with personal needs.
Parental Burnout: Recognize signs of parental burnout and strategies for prevention.

Sibling Relationships:

Sibling Dynamics: Understand the emotional dynamics between siblings and navigate conflicts.
Supporting Positive Relationships: Foster positive sibling relationships through communication and conflict resolution.

Blended Families:

Adjusting to New Roles: Navigate the emotional adjustments associated with blending families.
Effective Communication: Establish open communication to address challenges within blended family dynamics.

Crisis and Trauma:

Understanding Trauma:

Impact of Traumatic Events: Recognize the emotional impact of traumatic events on mental health.
Post-Traumatic Growth: Explore the concept of post-traumatic growth as a potential outcome of resilience.

SUPPORT NETWORKS AND POSTPARTUM CARE

The postpartum period, often referred to as the "fourth trimester," is a critical time for both physical and emotional recovery for new mothers. Adequate support networks and postpartum care play a pivotal role in ensuring the well-being of mothers during this transformative period.

The Significance of Support Networks:

Emotional Well-being:

Addressing Postpartum Blues: Understand the common emotional challenges faced by new mothers and the role of support in mitigating postpartum blues.
Preventing Postpartum Depression: Explore how strong support networks contribute to preventing and managing postpartum depression.

Physical Recovery:

Assisting with Daily Tasks: Recognize the impact of physical recovery on a new mother's ability to perform daily tasks and how support networks can aid in the process.

Encouraging Self-Care: Foster an environment where self-care is prioritized, allowing the mother to focus on her recovery.

Parenting Confidence:

Building Confidence: Support networks contribute to building parenting confidence by offering guidance, reassurance, and practical assistance.
Sharing Responsibilities: The distribution of parenting responsibilities within a support network helps reduce the burden on individual caregivers.

Relationship Dynamics:

Partner Support: Explore the pivotal role of partners in providing emotional and practical support during the postpartum period.
Extended Family Involvement: Understand how extended family members can contribute to creating a supportive environment for the new mother.

Roles within Support Networks:

Partner Support:

Emotional Encouragement: Partners can provide emotional encouragement, validate feelings, and actively participate in discussions about the new baby.

Assistance with Household Chores: Sharing household responsibilities allows the new mother to focus on her recovery and bonding with the baby.

Extended Family:

Practical Assistance: Grandparents, aunts, and uncles can offer practical assistance, such as meal preparation, grocery shopping, and childcare.
Providing Emotional Support: Extended family members contribute to emotional support, creating a nurturing environment for the new family.

Friends and Peers:

Emotional Understanding: Friends and peers can provide a different form of emotional understanding and often share relatable experiences.
Social Outings: Encouraging social outings helps the new mother maintain connections outside the immediate family.

Professional Support:

Healthcare Providers: Understand the role of healthcare providers, including doctors, nurses, and lactation consultants, in guiding the mother through physical recovery and addressing health concerns.
Mental Health Professionals: The support of mental health professionals is crucial for managing postpartum mental health issues.

Community Resources:

Parenting Classes: Engaging in parenting classes provides valuable information and connects new mothers with peers.
Postpartum Support Groups: Participating in support groups allows mothers to share experiences, seek advice, and build a sense of community.

Practical Steps for Building Support Networks:

Communication:

Open Dialogue: Encourage open communication within the support network to ensure everyone is on the same page.
Expressing Needs: New mothers should feel comfortable expressing their needs, preferences, and concerns to their support network.

Setting Boundaries:

Defining Boundaries: Establish clear boundaries with regard to visitors, chores, and responsibilities to prevent feelings of overwhelm.
Respecting Individual Space: Recognize the importance of individual space and downtime for the new mother.

Creating a Support Plan:

Preparation During Pregnancy: Develop a support plan during pregnancy, outlining the roles and responsibilities of each caregiver.
Postpartum Doula Services: Consider hiring postpartum doulas to provide professional assistance and guidance during the initial weeks.

Flexibility:

Adapting to Changing Needs: Recognize that the needs of the new mother may change, and support networks should be flexible in adapting to evolving circumstances.
Openness to Adjustments: Be open to adjusting roles and responsibilities based on the mother's preferences and well-being.

Self-Care Practices for New Mothers:

Rest and Sleep:

Prioritizing Rest: Encourage adequate rest by sharing nighttime duties and allowing the mother to nap during the day.
Creating a Sleep-Conducive Environment: Ensure a comfortable sleep environment to facilitate quality rest.

Nutrition:

Balanced Meals: Prepare nutritious meals or coordinate meal deliveries to support the mother's physical recovery.

Hydration: Encourage regular hydration, especially for breastfeeding mothers.

Physical Activity:

Gentle Exercises: Support the mother in engaging in gentle postpartum exercises, promoting physical well-being.
Outdoor Activities: Encourage short walks or spending time outdoors for a change of scenery and light physical activity.

Emotional Check-Ins:

Regular Conversations: Facilitate regular emotional check-ins to discuss feelings, concerns, and the overall emotional well-being of the new mother.
Acknowledging Achievements: Celebrate small achievements and milestones during the postpartum period.

Quality Time Alone:

Solo Activities: Encourage the mother to engage in activities she enjoys alone, providing moments of solitude and self-reflection.
Understanding Alone Time: Respect the need for occasional alone time and quiet moments for the mother to recharge.

Community Resources for Postpartum Care:

Postpartum Support Groups:

Online Communities: Explore online platforms and forums where mothers can connect with others experiencing similar postpartum challenges.
Local In-Person Groups: Join local support groups that facilitate face-to-face interactions and build a sense of community.

Parenting Classes:

Educational Programs: Participate in parenting classes that cover topics related to infant care, breastfeeding, and postpartum recovery.
Social Aspect: These classes provide opportunities to meet other parents, fostering a sense of camaraderie.

Home Visiting Programs:

Professional Assistance: Consider home visiting programs that provide professional support and guidance in the comfort of the mother's home.
Lactation Consultants: Seek the services of lactation consultants to address breastfeeding challenges and provide personalized guidance.

Telehealth Services:

Remote Counseling: Explore telehealth services for remote counseling sessions with mental health professionals.
Access to Healthcare Providers: Telehealth allows easy access to healthcare providers for postpartum check-ups and consultations.

PARENTING TIPS

BONDING WITH YOUR BABY

Bonding with your baby is a profound and transformative experience that lays the foundation for a lifelong relationship. From the early days of infancy through the various stages of childhood, fostering a strong emotional connection is essential for the well-being of both parent and child.

Understanding the Science of Bonding:

Oxytocin and the Bonding Hormone:

Role of Oxytocin: Explore the significance of oxytocin, often referred to as the "love hormone," in the bonding process.
Release Mechanisms: Understand the situations and activities that trigger oxytocin release in parents and infants.

Skin-to-Skin Contact:

Benefits of Skin-to-Skin: Examine the numerous advantages of skin-to-skin contact in the early postpartum period.
Promoting Bonding: Discover how this simple practice enhances bonding by creating a sense of warmth, security, and familiarity.

Eye Contact and Gaze:

Visual Connection: Learn about the importance of eye contact in building a visual connection between parent and baby.
Mutual Gaze: Understand how the mutual gaze enhances communication and emotional bonding.

Responsive Parenting:

Attunement to Cues: Explore the concept of responsive parenting, which involves recognizing and responding to your baby's cues promptly.
Building Trust: Understand how responsiveness fosters a sense of security and trust in the parent-child relationship.

Bonding During the Newborn Stage:

Caring for Your Newborn:

Feeding and Bonding: Examine the bonding opportunities during feeding, whether breastfeeding or bottle-feeding.
Diaper Changes and Bath Time: Understand how routine activities like diaper changes and bath time contribute to bonding.

Babywearing and Close Contact:

Benefits of Babywearing: Explore the advantages of using slings or carriers to keep your baby close throughout the day.
Multitasking and Bonding: Learn how babywearing allows parents to engage in various activities while maintaining physical closeness.

Reading and Singing:

Early Literacy and Bonding: Discover the benefits of reading and singing to your baby for language development and emotional connection.
Choosing Age-Appropriate Material: Select books and songs that align with your baby's developmental stage.

Creating a Calming Environment:

Soft Lighting and Soothing Sounds: Establish a calming environment with soft lighting and gentle sounds.
Infant Massage: Learn the art of infant massage to promote relaxation and bonding.

Bonding During Infancy and Toddlerhood:

Play and Exploration:

Floor Time Play: Engage in floor time play, allowing your baby to explore and interact with their surroundings.
Toy Selection: Choose age-appropriate toys that encourage exploration and sensory experiences.

Establishing Routines:

Consistent Bedtime Routines: Create bedtime routines that involve calming activities, fostering a sense of security.
Mealtime Connections: Make mealtimes a shared experience, providing opportunities for interaction and bonding.

Encouraging Independence:

Gradual Independence: Support your baby's growing sense of independence while maintaining a secure emotional connection.
Offering Choices: Encourage decision-making within age-appropriate boundaries to foster autonomy.

Social Interactions:

Playdates and Socialization: Arrange playdates and social interactions with other babies and parents.
Observing Social Cues: Help your baby understand social cues by modeling positive interactions and communication.

Parent-Child Bonding During Preschool and Early School Years:

Shared Activities:

Creative Arts: Engage in creative arts and crafts as a shared activity, fostering self-expression and bonding.
Outdoor Adventures: Explore the outdoors together through nature walks, visits to parks, and other outdoor adventures.

Building Emotional Intelligence:

Emotionally Supportive Conversations: Foster emotionally supportive conversations by validating your child's feelings and experiences.
Teaching Empathy: Encourage empathy by discussing others' perspectives and feelings.

Reading Together:

Interactive Reading: Transition to more interactive reading, where your child actively participates in storytelling.
Book Selection: Choose books that align with your child's interests and developmental stage.

Involvement in School Activities:

School Events Participation: Attend school events, performances, and activities to demonstrate your support and involvement.
Collaborating with Teachers: Establish positive relationships with your child's teachers to reinforce a sense of continuity between home and school.

Navigating Challenges and Special Circumstances:

Separation Anxiety:

Understanding Separation Anxiety: Recognize common signs of separation anxiety and implement strategies to ease transitions.
Gradual Separation: Gradually introduce short periods of separation to help your child build confidence.

Blended Families and Sibling Dynamics:

Blended Family Bonding: Foster a sense of belonging and inclusion within blended families through open communication and shared activities.
Sibling Relationships: Encourage positive sibling relationships by promoting cooperation, empathy, and conflict resolution.

Special Circumstances:

Preterm Birth and NICU Stay: Address the unique challenges of bonding after preterm birth or a NICU stay.
Adoption: Explore strategies to build a strong parent-child bond in the context of adoption.

Maintaining a Strong Connection During Adolescence:

Open Communication:

Encouraging Dialogue: Create a supportive environment for open communication, allowing your adolescent to express their thoughts and feelings.
Active Listening: Practice active listening to strengthen the parent-child connection.

Respecting Independence:

Balancing Independence: Acknowledge and respect your adolescent's growing need for independence while maintaining a supportive role.
Negotiating Boundaries: Engage in open discussions to negotiate age-appropriate boundaries.

Shared Interests:

Identifying Common Interests: Explore shared hobbies or interests to strengthen the emotional connection.
Quality Time: Prioritize quality time together, even as schedules become busier.

Practical Tips for Bonding at Every Stage:

Quality Time or Quantity Time:

Presence and Engagement: Emphasize the importance of being present and engaged during quality time, even if it's limited.
Meaningful Connections: Create meaningful connections through intentional interactions and shared experiences.

Adapting to Your Child's Needs:

Flexibility in Parenting Styles: Be adaptable in your parenting approach, considering the individual needs and temperament of your child.
Parenting Challenges: Address challenges with flexibility, seeking solutions that align with your child's development.

BALANCING WORK AND FAMILY

Balancing the demands of a career with the responsibilities of family life is a complex and dynamic challenge that many individuals face. Striking a harmonious balance between work and family is crucial for maintaining overall well-being and satisfaction.

Understanding the Dynamics:

Changing Work Landscape:

Evolution of Work Structures: Explore how the modern work environment has evolved, with remote work, flexible hours, and alternative work arrangements becoming more prevalent.
Impact on Work-Life Balance: Understand how these changes influence the dynamics of balancing work and family life.

Importance of Work-Life Balance:

Physical and Mental Health: Delve into the implications of maintaining a healthy work-life balance on both physical and mental well-being.

Productivity and Job Satisfaction: Explore the positive impact of balance on workplace productivity and job satisfaction.

Challenges in Balancing Work and Family:

Time Constraints: Understand the time pressures that can arise from competing demands between work and family.

Guilt and Stress: Examine the emotional challenges, including guilt and stress, that individuals may experience when trying to balance these two critical aspects of life.

Strategies for Balancing Work and Family:

Time Management:

Prioritization Techniques: Explore effective prioritization methods to allocate time efficiently to work and family responsibilities.

Setting Boundaries: Establish clear boundaries to protect personal time and prevent work from encroaching on family life.

Flexible Work Arrangements:

Remote Work: Examine the benefits and challenges of remote work, providing flexibility that allows individuals to better manage family commitments.
Part-Time or Flexible Hours: Explore part-time work or flexible hours as options to strike a balance between work and family.

Effective Communication:

Open Dialogue with Employers: Encourage open communication with employers about family commitments and the potential need for flexibility.
Negotiating Work Expectations: Negotiate realistic expectations and workloads to align with personal responsibilities.

Setting Realistic Goals:

Achievable Objectives: Establish realistic short-term and long-term goals, acknowledging the need for balance in various life domains.
Balancing Ambition and Well-being: Understand the delicate balance between professional ambition and personal well-being.

Coping with Parenthood and Career Advancement:

Parental Leave Policies:

Understanding Parental Leave: Explore the importance of parental leave policies for new parents.

Balancing Return to Work: Discuss strategies for transitioning back to work after parental leave.

Childcare Support:

Choosing Childcare Options: Evaluate various childcare options, including daycare, nannies, or family assistance.
Family Support Networks: Leverage family support networks to share childcare responsibilities.

Career Advancement Strategies:

Mentorship and Sponsorship: Explore the role of mentorship and sponsorship in career advancement for both men and women.
Negotiation Skills: Develop negotiation skills to assertively communicate career aspirations while considering family needs.

Workplace Policies and Initiatives:

Supportive Workplace Culture: Assess the importance of workplace cultures that support both career growth and work-life balance.
Wellness Programs: Explore the benefits of workplace wellness programs that cater to the holistic needs of employees.

Practical Tips for Balancing Work and Family Life:

Creating a Family Calendar:

Visualizing Commitments: Develop a family calendar that visualizes work and family commitments, helping to plan and allocate time effectively.
Shared Schedules: Ensure family members are aware of each other's schedules to avoid conflicts and encourage mutual support.

Quality over Quantity Time:

Focused Interactions: Emphasize the importance of quality time over quantity, fostering meaningful interactions with family members.
Mindful Presence: Be present in the moment during family time, minimizing distractions from work-related concerns.

Prioritizing Self-Care:

Physical and Mental Well-being: Prioritize self-care practices, including exercise, proper nutrition, and adequate sleep.
Setting Personal Boundaries: Establish personal boundaries to prevent burnout and maintain overall health.

Delegating Responsibilities:

Sharing Household Duties: Collaborate with family members to share household responsibilities, preventing one individual from feeling overwhelmed.
Outsourcing Tasks: Consider outsourcing tasks such as house cleaning or grocery shopping to save time and reduce stress.

Navigating Challenges and Coping Mechanisms:

Handling Guilt and Stress:

Accepting Imperfections: Acknowledge that achieving a perfect balance is challenging, and imperfections are a natural part of the process.
Coping Mechanisms: Develop coping mechanisms to handle guilt and stress effectively, such as mindfulness and stress reduction techniques.

Parental Roles and Expectations:

Reassessing Traditional Roles: Challenge traditional gender roles and expectations regarding parenting responsibilities.
Equal Partnership: Strive for an equal partnership in parenting, with shared responsibilities for childcare and household duties.

Building a Support Network:

Connecting with Other Parents: Engage with other parents facing similar challenges through support groups or social networks.
Professional and Peer Support: Seek support from colleagues, mentors, or peers who understand the complexities of balancing work and family.

Long-Term Strategies for Sustainable Balance:

Career Planning and Flexibility:

Strategic Career Planning: Engage in strategic career planning that aligns with personal and family goals.
Adapting to Changing Priorities: Be flexible in adapting career goals to changing life priorities and stages.

Life Transitions and Reassessments:

Regular Reassessments: Periodically reassess work and family priorities to align with evolving life stages.
Navigating Transitions: Develop strategies for navigating major life transitions, such as a change in career or relocation.

Cultivating Resilience:

Embracing Resilience: Cultivate resilience to navigate challenges and setbacks, recognizing them as opportunities for growth.

Learning from Experiences: Reflect on past experiences to identify lessons and strategies for overcoming obstacles.

Creating a Family-Friendly Work Culture:

Employer Initiatives:

Flexible Work Policies: Advocate for flexible work policies and initiatives that support a family-friendly work culture.
Telecommuting Options: Explore telecommuting options and remote work opportunities to enhance flexibility.

Promoting Work-Life Balance:

Encouraging Boundaries: Encourage a workplace culture that respects and promotes personal boundaries.
Wellness Programs: Implement wellness programs that address both physical and mental health needs.

CHILDPROOFING AND SAFETY MEASURES

Childproofing your home is a crucial aspect of parenting that involves identifying potential hazards and implementing safety measures to create a secure environment for your child. Ensuring a safe space for your child is essential for fostering healthy growth and curiosity while minimizing the risk of accidents and injuries.

Understanding Child Development and Safety:

Curiosity and Exploration:

Curiosity in Early Childhood: Explore how a child's innate curiosity drives them to explore their surroundings.
Developmental Stages: Understand age-appropriate behaviors and developmental stages that impact a child's interaction with the environment.

Common Household Dangers:

Choking Hazards: Identify common household items that pose a choking risk, especially for infants and toddlers.
Falls and Injury Risks: Recognize potential fall hazards, sharp edges, and other factors contributing to the risk of injuries.

Safety Considerations for Different Age Groups:

Infant Safety: Focus on measures to protect infants, such as safe sleep practices and baby-proofing specific areas.
Toddler Safety: Implement safety measures tailored to the increased mobility and curiosity of toddlers.

Preschooler Safety: Adjust childproofing strategies as children become more independent and capable of reaching higher areas.

Childproofing Strategies for Every Room:

Kitchen Safety:

Cabinet Locks: Install cabinet locks to prevent access to potentially harmful items such as cleaning supplies and sharp objects.
Stove Guards: Implement stove guards to protect against burns and scalds.

Living Room and Play Area:

Anchor Furniture: Secure heavy furniture and appliances to the wall to prevent tip-overs.
Cushion Sharp Edges: Use edge guards or corner protectors on furniture with sharp edges.

Bedroom Safety:

Safe Sleep Practices: Follow safe sleep guidelines for infants, including using a firm mattress and avoiding soft bedding.
Window Cord Safety: Install cordless window coverings to eliminate the risk of strangulation.

Bathroom Safety:

Secure Medications and Cleaning Products: Store medications and cleaning products out of reach or in locked cabinets.
Anti-Slip Measures: Use non-slip mats in the bathtub to prevent slips and falls.

Stair Safety:

Stair Gates: Install safety gates at the top and bottom of stairs to restrict access.
Secure Railings: Ensure that stair railings are secure and meet safety standards.

Outdoor Safety:

Fence the Yard: Install a fence around the yard to prevent accidental wandering.
Supervision Guidelines: Establish guidelines for outdoor play and supervise children when playing in outdoor areas.

Essential Childproofing Products:

Safety Gates:

Types of Safety Gates: Explore the various types of safety gates suitable for stairs, doorways, and wider openings.
Installation Tips: Follow proper installation guidelines to ensure gates are securely in place.

Outlet Covers and Plug Protectors:

Outlet Cover Options: Choose outlet covers or plug protectors to prevent children from inserting objects into electrical outlets.
Using Tamper-Resistant Outlets: Consider installing tamper-resistant outlets for added safety.

Cabinet and Drawer Locks:

Types of Locks: Implement different types of cabinet and drawer locks based on the specific needs of each area.
Installation Techniques: Ensure proper installation to effectively secure cabinets and drawers.

Corner and Edge Protectors:

Materials and Designs: Select corner and edge protectors made of soft materials to cushion potential impact.
Application on Furniture: Apply protectors to sharp corners and edges of furniture, countertops, and other surfaces.

Window and Blind Cord Safety:

Cordless Window Coverings: Opt for cordless window coverings to eliminate the risk of strangulation.
Securing Blind Cords: Use cord cleats or wind-ups to secure blind cords out of a child's reach.

Furniture Anchors:

Securing Heavy Furniture: Anchor heavy furniture, bookshelves, and appliances to the wall to prevent tipping.
Installation Steps: Follow proper installation steps to ensure stability.

Childproofing for Different Developmental Stages:

Infant Safety Measures:

Safe Sleep Practices: Implement guidelines for safe sleep, including placing infants on their backs in a crib with a firm mattress.
Monitoring Temperature: Maintain a comfortable room temperature and avoid overdressing infants.

Toddler and Preschooler Safety Considerations:

Secure Furniture and TVs: Anchor furniture and secure TVs to prevent tip-overs.
Supervision and Boundaries: Provide constant supervision and establish clear boundaries for play areas.

School-Age Child Safety:

Teaching Safety Rules: Educate school-age children about safety rules, including road safety and fire escape plans.

Cyber Safety: Address digital safety concerns, including internet usage and online interactions.

Educational Approaches to Safety:

Safety Education:

Age-Appropriate Lessons: Provide age-appropriate safety lessons, teaching children about potential dangers and how to avoid them.
Role-Playing Scenarios: Use role-playing scenarios to help children practice safety behaviors.

Emergency Preparedness:

Fire Drills: Conduct regular fire drills at home, emphasizing evacuation routes and meeting points.
Emergency Contacts: Teach children how to dial emergency numbers and memorize important contact information.

Regular Safety Assessments and Updates:

Regular Inspections:

Scheduled Assessments: Conduct periodic safety assessments of the home, focusing on potential hazards.
Updating Childproofing Measures: Update childproofing measures as the child grows and new hazards emerge.

Consulting Professionals:

Home Safety Inspections: Consider professional home safety inspections to identify hidden hazards.
Healthcare Provider Guidance: Consult with healthcare providers for guidance on age-appropriate safety measures.

Promoting Independence and Responsibility:

Teaching Safety Awareness:

Gradual Independence: Foster gradual independence by teaching children safety awareness and self-regulation.
Empowering Decision-Making: Encourage responsible decision-making regarding safety and risk assessment.

Positive Reinforcement:

Celebrating Safe Behaviors: Use positive reinforcement to celebrate and reward safe behaviors.
Encouraging Communication: Create an open dialogue where children feel comfortable discussing safety concerns.

childproofing and implementing safety measures in your home are fundamental aspects of responsible parenting. By understanding the developmental stages of your child, recognizing potential hazards, and employing practical childproofing strategies, you can create a safe and nurturing environment for your child's growth.

FINANCIAL PLANNING

BUDGETING FOR A NEW ARRIVAL

Welcoming a new arrival into your family is an exciting and transformative experience, but it also comes with financial responsibilities that require careful planning. Effective financial planning not only provides stability but also allows you to focus on the joys of parenthood without unnecessary stress.

Anticipating Pregnancy Costs:

Prenatal Care Expenses:

Health Insurance Coverage: Understand your health insurance coverage for prenatal care, including doctor visits, ultrasounds, and screenings.
Out-of-Pocket Costs: Be prepared for potential out-of-pocket expenses related to copayments and deductibles.

Maternity Clothing and Essentials:

Budgeting for Clothing: Allocate funds for maternity clothing as your body changes during pregnancy.
Essential Supplies: Plan for the purchase of maternity essentials such as prenatal vitamins, body pillows, and comfortable footwear.

Preparing the Nursery:

Furniture and Decor: Budget for nursery furniture, decor, and essentials like a crib, changing table, and storage.
Painting and Safety Measures: Account for any painting or safety measures required for the nursery.

Childbirth Classes and Resources:

Educational Classes: Consider the cost of childbirth education classes to prepare for labor and delivery.
Books and Online Resources: Budget for relevant books, apps, or online resources to supplement your knowledge.

Building a Baby Budget:

Setting Up a Baby Fund:

Emergency Fund: Establish or replenish an emergency fund to cover unexpected expenses.
Baby-Specific Savings: Create a separate savings account specifically earmarked for baby-related costs.

Reviewing Current Expenses:

Budget Assessment: Conduct a comprehensive review of your current household budget.
Identifying Non-Essentials: Identify non-essential expenses that could be trimmed or cut temporarily.

Health Insurance Considerations:

Coverage for the Baby: Review health insurance policies to understand coverage for the baby after birth.
Pediatric Care Costs: Anticipate costs related to pediatric care and vaccinations.

Workplace Benefits and Parental Leave:

Parental Leave Policies: Understand parental leave policies at your workplace, including paid and unpaid options.
Access to Benefits: Determine access to workplace benefits like flexible spending accounts (FSAs) or health savings accounts (HSAs).

Budgeting During Maternity and Paternity Leave:

Assessing Income Changes:

Temporary Income Reduction: Plan for a temporary reduction in income during maternity or paternity leave.
Calculating Paid Leave: If applicable, calculate the income received during paid leave.

Prioritizing Essential Expenses:

Identifying Priorities: Prioritize essential expenses, such as mortgage or rent, utilities, and groceries.
Temporary Adjustments: Temporarily adjust non-essential spending to accommodate the reduced income.

Utilizing Workplace Benefits:

Paid Time Off: If available, use paid time off or vacation days to supplement income.
Short-Term Disability: Understand short-term disability benefits, if applicable, and how they can contribute to income during leave.

Exploring Government Assistance Programs:

Family and Medical Leave Act (FMLA): Determine eligibility for FMLA, which provides job protection during leave.
State and Local Programs: Explore state or local programs that may offer additional support or benefits.

Preparing for Ongoing Baby Expenses:

Baby Gear and Supplies:

Creating a Registry: Utilize baby registries to share essential needs with friends and family.
Second-Hand Options: Consider purchasing gently used baby items to save on costs.

Childcare Costs:

Daycare or Nanny Services: Research local childcare options and estimate associated costs.

Flexible Work Arrangements: Explore flexible work arrangements or options for shared childcare responsibilities.

Feeding and Diapering Expenses:

Breastfeeding vs. Formula Costs: Compare the costs of breastfeeding and formula feeding, including related supplies.
Diapering Choices: Evaluate the costs associated with disposable versus cloth diapers.

Education and Future Planning:

College Savings: Consider starting a college savings fund for your child's future education.
Life Insurance Planning: Assess life insurance options to provide financial security for your family.

Smart Shopping Strategies:

Sales, Discounts, and Coupons:

Timing Purchases: Take advantage of sales, discounts, and seasonal promotions when making baby-related purchases.
Coupon Utilization: Use coupons or participate in loyalty programs to save on essential items.

Bulk Purchases and Gift Considerations:

Buying in Bulk: Consider bulk purchases for items with a longer shelf life, such as diapers and wipes.
Gift Suggestions: Share practical gift suggestions with friends and family to receive items you truly need.

Second-Hand and Hand-Me-Downs:

Thrifting for Baby Items: Explore thrift stores or consignment shops for affordable baby clothing and gear.
Hand-Me-Downs: Accept hand-me-downs from friends or family for items like baby clothes, furniture, and toys.

Financial Planning Beyond the Newborn Stage:

Ongoing Education and Extracurriculars:

Planning for Activities: Anticipate costs associated with extracurricular activities, classes, and educational materials.
Prioritizing Interests: Prioritize activities based on your child's interests and your budget constraints.

Child-Proofing the Home:

Upgrading Safety Measures: As your child grows, revisit childproofing measures to adapt to new safety concerns.
Assessing Developmental Needs: Adjust the home environment to meet your child's changing developmental needs.

Reviewing and Adjusting the Budget:

Regular Budget Reviews: Conduct regular reviews of your budget to ensure alignment with changing family needs.
Adjusting Priorities: Be flexible in adjusting financial priorities as your child grows and family dynamics change.

Investing in Your Child's Future:

Education Savings Accounts (ESAs) and 529 Plans:

Setting Up College Funds: Explore ESAs or 529 plans to save for your child's higher education.
Contributions and Tax Benefits: Understand contribution limits and potential tax benefits associated with these accounts.

Teaching Financial Literacy:

Age-Appropriate Lessons: Introduce age-appropriate financial lessons to help your child develop sound money management skills.
Savings Habits: Encourage savings habits by involving your child in setting aside money for specific goals.

Emergency Fund for Unforeseen Expenses:

Maintaining an Emergency Fund: Continue to prioritize and maintain an emergency fund for unforeseen expenses.

PLANNING FOR PARENTAL LEAVE

Welcoming a new addition to the family is an exciting and transformative experience, and planning for parental leave is a crucial aspect of this journey. Effective planning ensures a smooth transition into parenthood, allowing individuals to embrace the joys of this new chapter while maintaining financial stability and professional growth.

Understanding Parental Leave Policies:

Employer Policies:

Reviewing Company Policies: Understand parental leave policies provided by your employer, including duration, eligibility criteria, and benefits.
Documentation Requirements: Familiarize yourself with any required documentation or notification processes for requesting parental leave.

Government Regulations:

Family and Medical Leave Act (FMLA): Explore the provisions of FMLA, a federal law that provides eligible employees with up to 12 weeks of unpaid leave for certain family and medical reasons.

State and Local Regulations: Be aware of additional parental leave regulations that may exist at the state or local level, providing extended benefits or different conditions.

Negotiating Leave Terms:

Open Communication with Employers: Establish open communication with employers to discuss leave terms, including start and end dates, part-time options, or remote work arrangements.
Flexible Scheduling: Negotiate flexible scheduling options if needed, such as a gradual return to full-time work.

Financial Planning During Parental Leave:

Understanding Paid Leave:

Paid Parental Leave Policies: Review employer policies regarding paid parental leave, including any stipulations or limitations.
Supplemental Income: Understand how paid leave interacts with other benefits, like sick leave or vacation days, to supplement income.

Short-Term Disability Benefits:

Exploring Disability Coverage: Some parental leaves may qualify for short-term disability benefits; explore the eligibility criteria and coverage provided.

Understanding Duration: Determine the duration and amount of disability benefits, which may partially replace lost income during parental leave.

Accrued Time Off and Vacation Days:

Using Accrued Time Off: Consider using accrued time off or vacation days to extend the duration of paid leave.
Discussing Options with HR: Consult with Human Resources to understand policies regarding the use of accrued time off.

Unpaid Leave Considerations:

Budgeting for Unpaid Time: Plan for the financial impact of any unpaid parental leave, including adjustments to the household budget.
Emergency Fund Usage: Utilize emergency funds as a financial safety net during periods of unpaid leave.

Work-Life Balance and Family Time:

Setting Realistic Expectations:

Establishing Boundaries: Communicate and set boundaries with colleagues regarding work expectations during parental leave.
Realistic Personal Goals: Set realistic personal goals for balancing family time, self-care, and work responsibilities.

Quality Family Time:

Prioritizing Family Activities: Plan and prioritize quality family time during parental leave to bond with the new addition and support your partner.
Creating Memorable Moments: Engage in activities that create lasting memories, fostering a positive family dynamic.

Self-Care Practices:

Prioritizing Well-being: Emphasize the importance of self-care for both parents during parental leave.
Identifying Stressors: Recognize potential stressors and proactively address them to maintain mental and emotional well-being.

Maintaining Connections:

Connecting with the Child: Foster connections with the newborn by actively participating in caregiving responsibilities.
Staying Connected with Partners: Communicate openly with your partner, ensuring shared responsibilities and mutual support.

Planning the Return to Work:

Transitioning Back to Work:

Gradual Return: Explore options for a gradual return to work, such as part-time schedules or flexible hours.
Re-establishing Work Routines: Plan for re-establishing work routines while considering family needs.

Childcare Arrangements:

Researching Childcare Options: Begin researching and securing childcare arrangements well in advance.
Choosing the Right Provider: Consider factors such as proximity, safety, and reputation when selecting a childcare provider.

Communicating with Employers:

Return-to-Work Plan: Develop a return-to-work plan in collaboration with your employer, outlining expectations and any necessary accommodations.
Work Schedule Negotiation: If needed, negotiate modifications to your work schedule that align with family responsibilities.

Managing Work Stress:

Open Dialogue with Supervisors: Maintain open communication with supervisors about workload expectations and potential stressors.
Utilizing Resources: Explore workplace resources such as Employee Assistance Programs (EAPs) for additional support.

Maintaining Career Growth and Development:

Professional Development Goals:

Setting Career Objectives: Establish short-term and long-term professional development goals.
Revisiting Career Plans: Periodically revisit and adjust career plans to align with evolving family needs.

Networking and Mentorship:

Maintaining Professional Connections: Stay connected with professional networks and colleagues during parental leave.
Seeking Mentorship: Consider seeking mentorship to navigate career challenges and transitions.

Advocating for Workplace Flexibility:

Promoting Flexible Work Policies: Advocate for workplace flexibility and family-friendly policies that support a healthy work-life balance.
Participating in Employee Resource Groups: Join employee resource groups or networks that focus on work-life balance and parenting.

Long-Term Career Planning:

Strategic Career Planning:

Aligning Career Goals: Align career goals with long-term family aspirations, considering factors such as relocation or career changes.

Professional Development Opportunities: Seek out professional development opportunities that complement both career growth and family life.

Navigating Career Transitions:

Considering Career Transitions: Be open to considering career transitions that align better with evolving family priorities.

Balancing Personal and Professional Goals: Strive for a balance that accommodates both personal and professional aspirations.

Cultivating a Supportive Work Environment:

Encouraging Family-Friendly Policies: Encourage the adoption of family-friendly policies in the workplace to support employees at different life stages.

Participating in Workplace Initiatives: Participate in workplace initiatives that promote work-life balance, employee well-being, and inclusivity.

planning for parental leave is a multifaceted process that involves understanding leave policies, financial planning, and maintaining a healthy work-life balance. By approaching parental leave with thoughtful consideration and proactive planning, individuals can successfully navigate the challenges of parenthood while continuing to thrive in their professional careers. The key is to strike a balance that allows for meaningful family time, self-care, and sustained career growth, creating a fulfilling and harmonious life journey.

www.ingramcontent.com/pod-product-compliance
Lightning Source LLC
Chambersburg PA
CBHW070834250726
48662CB00003B/1219